Breakthrough Babies

An IVF pioneer's tale of creating life
against all odds

by
Simon Fishel

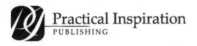

Practical Inspiration
PUBLISHING

First published in Great Britain by Practical Inspiration Publishing, 2019

ISBN 978-1-78860-073-6

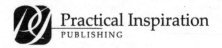

Practical Inspiration
PUBLISHING

In loving memory of Devra Grugel (Cohen), whose love of life and unique positivity for the world around her was taken from us far too early. Her memory and the paths she lit for so many will forever burn brightly in our hearts.

Contents

List of Figures

Foreword

The 'beacon of triumph' that Louise Brown's birth represented as the first test tube baby set a pattern for media coverage of the revolution in human reproduction for the next forty years. Her arrival led a world exclusive on the front page of the *Daily Mail* on 25 July 1978, where she was billed as 'the lovely Louise', and was unequivocally a turning point for childless couples. She burst through a wall of secrecy that surrounded the research, rightly so given the opposition from some in the medical establishment that marked not just the early days of technical achievements in fertility treatment, but the heated debates over the ethics and regulation that would follow.

The drama and controversies were a gift to journalists. Not only did we have the excitement of fast-moving scientific innovation but the narrative of hopelessness behind the human stories which were the heart of the matter. Simon Fishel's memoirs give us a first-hand account of a medical science pioneer in at the start – his remarkable contribution began with research in the field before Louise Brown was born – and he has yet to complete the journey. He has unfinished business to do in transforming women's lives after the menopause which may even extend their childbearing potential. Yet the vital element throughout is his understanding and empathy with the pioneering patients who took the risks along with the scientists.

Fishel's belief is that 'every baby is a miracle' in fertility treatment. It's also compelling copy for the media as shown by the tenor of coverage during the first twenty years of IVF milestones. Journalists were competing with each other for the next first birth occurring after the slightest advance in an esoteric technique. Broadly speaking, these were good news stories but with the spice of doom-laden warnings from critics that doctors were 'playing God'. The hostile environment created by acknowledged dilemmas and personal rivalries was a fascinating backdrop, but nothing that would get in the way of a good story. The public appetite for the joy of lives transformed by scientists who admitted they were working in the dark was insatiable. The paradox that dogged IVF research – proving a technique was safe in humans before using it – may have kept doctors awake at night. But it took centre stage for reporters only when the regulators, lawyers and ethicists formulated rules that stood in the way of the hopes and dreams of people prepared to do anything to have a baby.

Fishel's driving force has always been to 'work at the limits of what's possible'. It's no wonder the media responded to his willingness to seize the window of opportunity and circumvent the hasty erection of barriers to human endeavour. I remember writing the splash in the *Daily Mail* on 7 September 1992 which invited readers to 'Meet James the First'. Once again, Fishel had pushed the cutting edge of IVF treatment to the maximum for people who had run out of hope. His rollercoaster ride through forty years of scientific advances provides a microcosm of a revolution in human conception taking place in laboratories, hospitals, and universities around the world. Yet at the same time he was battling demons that could have taken him down, from the threat of bankruptcy to having a gun held to his head by a maverick colleague, with a resilience that is genuinely admirable.

The quest for perfect embryos inevitably escalated into ethical and legal controversies over what some regarded as the ultimate destination – perfect people. The media relished the new challenge, far more than the desperate individuals caught up in personal tragedies played out on the public stage. Many of these stories ended in despair. At the same time IVF was re-defining family life at a pace that seems even more breathtaking looking back. The social acceptance of the implications of a procession of technical acronyms such as SUZI, ICSI, PGD, CGH, has accompanied a broad tolerance of the means to end the misery of infertility which went on to embrace much wider issues such as the sex selection of embryos. As head of CARE, the largest IVF group in the UK, Fishel can rightly claim to be in the vanguard of a global movement that's led to the birth of eight million IVF babies so far. But the story doesn't end here for him or the media. Science has reached a point in human history where medical intervention is more efficient than nature in human conception. But it is also inextricably bound into the threads of advances in DNA technology that made possible the cloning of Dolly the sheep and could even result in predictably reliable human cloning. It's a legacy to ponder.

Jenny Hope
Award-winning journalist[1]

---

[1] Mind Journalist of the Year 2009, Recipient of the annual ICRF/ Cancer Research Fund Distinction in Reporting Award 2000, Millennium Nurse Nursing in the Media awards Joint National Media Winner 1999, BMA Medical Journalist of the Year 1998, British Dental Health Foundation Journalist of the Year 1991, Medical Journalist's Association Awards Winner, Royal College of Nursing Journalist of the Year

Special Note

When I was born in 1978, the impact was felt all around the world. Robert Edwards and Patrick Steptoe had achieved the success they had been craving for many years. For my mum Lesley and dad John, it was the dream ending to a struggle to have a child that had lasted almost ten years. IVF had worked at the first try for Mum and she just wanted to go home and enjoy her baby. She could not have imagined at that moment how Assisted Reproductive Technology would develop to what we see today.

Soon Edwards and Steptoe had established the first IVF clinic, Bourn Hall, near Cambridge. My mum had her second treatment there and it worked first time again – bringing my sister Natalie into the world. She was only the fortieth IVF baby in the world, and Simon Fishel was part of the team that created her.

I enjoyed many happy hours at Bourn Hall as a child, meeting the ever-growing IVF family which is now in the millions and spread worldwide. I saw first-hand how Simon, and others like him, continued to push the boundaries and develop new techniques so that today more and more people can find a solution to their fertility problems. It is only by having pioneers that medical science can progress.

We need good regulation of fertility treatment but above all we need to have trust in the doctors working on taking fertility treatment to new levels. They need the freedom to try out new things – as Bob Edwards did to create me. I hope that by reading this story others are inspired to push the boundaries. Long may Simon Fishel continue with his work.

Louise Brown,
The world's first 'test tube baby'

Chapter 1

Nobody Said It Would Be Easy

'Oh, what a tangled web we weave, when first we practise to conceive.'
Don Herold, US humourist

It was my son Matt's first day at school many years ago, and his teacher gathered her apprehensive pupils around her. 'Let's get to know each other', she said. 'What do your mums and dads do for a living?' A forest of eager hands shot up. When it came to Matt's turn, his answer was obvious.

My dad makes babies.

He was right. As an in vitro fertilisation (IVF) practitioner, researcher, and teacher for forty years, it's what I do and what I've always done. It's what I plan on sticking with for a while longer, too. To me every baby is a miracle and there's no experience more amazing and rewarding than seeing it at its earliest stage – as a sperm and an egg. Most are conceived without difficulty but for those who aren't, my work revolves around giving those cells a vital nudge along the way. In doing so, I've been lucky enough to see with my own eyes the spectacular process of cell division that normally happens hidden from view, inside the human body.

I'm always aware, though, that while I can put sperm and egg together, what happens afterwards is driven by a force beyond my control. Eventually the resulting baby will become part of a family – the building block of our society. In this way, IVF plays a role far beyond the medical. It's responsible for bringing joy and delight to thousands of couples, for giving children to those who don't fit society's model of a 'normal' parent, and more recently, for eliminating genetic diseases from a family line.

At the beginning of my career I worked closely with Robert (Bob) Edwards and Patrick Steptoe, the 'fathers' of IVF, as they pioneered the technology that became known as 'test tube babies'. This gave me a front row seat at the theatre of elations and frustrations at that exciting time. Since then I've gone on to develop yet more innovative and effective ways of giving babies to infertile people, helping to spread IVF technology around the world. This is important, because although the creation of IVF was a ground-breaking achievement, there have been many more significant discoveries in human embryology since Louise Brown – the first test tube baby – was born in 1978. Geneticists, physiologists, doctors, and patients – all have been pioneers who've helped develop this work in addition to scientists like myself. While Bob and Patrick opened the door to a collaborative process of discovery, what came afterwards was a continuation of their greatness.

But here's a thought: in regulated countries such as the UK, IVF couldn't be invented today. The regulatory bodies that govern medical research would forbid it. This was confirmed recently by a senior member of our own regulatory organisation, the Human Fertilisation and Embryology Association (HFEA), who told me that if Patrick and Bob had been practising in a modern climate, they would have been stopped a long time before Louise Brown was born, and Patrick would have been reported to the General Medical Council. Of course regulation is necessary, but innovation in science involves taking risks. When we leap into the unknown it goes without saying that we don't know what the exact outcome will be; as long as all parties know this and the aim is worthwhile, this is something we have to accept.

To push back the boundaries of medical science takes courage and a dogged willingness to keep going against all odds. These are qualities Bob and Patrick had in abundance during their ten-year struggle to make IVF work, and led to the creation of a technology that has been world changing. It's also been highly criticised. It's easy to forget how controversial it once was to fertilise a human egg in a test tube; it was a practice viewed with the utmost suspicion. The easiest way of gaining a feel for it is to look at the commentary around cloning today: it's 'playing God' and 'taking science too far'. That's how it was with human IVF when I first started working in it in 1980 – and to a certain extent still is now – because science will always speed ahead more quickly than people's minds can accept. This aversion to risk has led to what I call the paradox of IVF: to develop something innovative that will help people in a way that's not been done before, we need to do new things. These new things may not work, and they might even offend some people. The regulator doesn't like that uncertainty. So what to do? Undertake research to prove ahead of time everything's fine? But surely that's what research is for in the first place? You can see the catch-22 situation I've worked in for most of my career.

The year of writing, 2018 – shortly after the fortieth anniversary of Louise Brown's birth in Oldham, UK – has been a special one for me as it's prompted some reflection on how far IVF has progressed since those days. Much of the journey has been a fascinating one, with many a 'what if?' along the way. What if IVF had been as heavily controlled then as it is now? What if I'd not later discovered a way to help 40 per cent more infertile couples to have babies? What if I'd been allowed to use many of the techniques I developed, instead of being prevented from doing so by regulation? What would be the outcome today?

I could also ask why I've devoted my life to this thing called IVF. It's because I was, and still am, fascinated by the phenomenal ability our cells have to reproduce, and because I love helping people to become fulfilled. To realise the great contribution to humanity I believe IVF is capable of, I've had to push ahead with new research without knowing ahead of time if it will work, and in the face of fierce opposition. It's taken all my irrepressible enthusiasm and energy to keep going despite the numerous setbacks detailed in this book. I admit I've had more failures than successes, but that's part of the work I'm in – it's not for the faint hearted.

On the rare occasions on which I've struggled to motivate myself to keep going against all odds, I'm energised by what JF Kennedy said to rally support for the work that ultimately led to the first moon landing:

> We choose to go to the Moon in this decade and do
> the other things, not because they are easy, but because
> they are hard; because that goal will serve to organise
> and measure the best of our energies and skills, because
> that challenge is one that we are willing to accept, one
> we are unwilling to postpone, and one we intend to
> win. (John F. Kennedy. Speech, Rice Stadium, Houston,
> Texas, 12 September 1962)

I love these words, not because I liken myself to someone of
the status of a US president, but because I too have never been
one to shrink from a challenge simply because it's hard. If I
think the outcome is worthwhile I'll move heaven and earth
to achieve it, even if it involves me almost going bankrupt,
being pilloried in the press, or having a gun put to my head.
These things really happened! In the following chapters you'll
learn more about them, and also discover how IVF began at the
world's very first clinic, how I took that work forward to help
thousands of people have the babies they wanted, and how I
almost lost everything in the process.

Enjoy the ride.

Chapter 2

Bourn Hall: The World's First IVF Clinic

1980–1985

My IVF career was born, at the age of 27, in two simultaneous locations: a wood-panelled office at Cambridge University and the more prosaic environs of the portacabins at Bourn Hall. Not that the hall wasn't a lovely building – it was a magnificent, 400-year-old house in the middle of the Cambridgeshire countryside surrounded by rolling lawns and gardens – but the clinical facilities necessarily took second place to the needs of patients, who were welcomed and consulted in the main house. The year was 1980, Abba were cruising the charts, and Bob Edwards had invited me to join him there as his Deputy Scientific Director. Patrick Steptoe, Bob's co-pioneer and colleague from Oldham, was Medical Director, and John Webster, who'd assisted with the birth of Louise Brown, was appointed Deputy Medical Director. Supporting us was Jean Purdy as Laboratory Assistant; she'd played a pivotal role in helping Bob and Patrick during their time in Oldham and was instrumental in setting up Bourn Hall. In fact, in later years Bob was adamant she be recognised by including her name with his and Patrick's on the blue plaque commemorating the clinic where Louise was conceived.

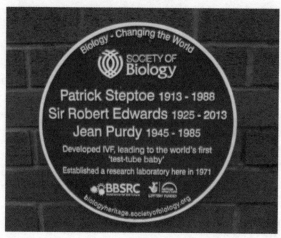

Figure 2.1: Wall plaque at Dr Kershaw's Hospice in Oldham

Bourn Hall was a bold venture. In the two-year gap between Louise being born and the hall opening, only two more IVF babies had come into the world. One was Alastair MacDonald who was conceived in the same Oldham hospital a few months after Louise, and another in Australia in 1980. There was also a baby in India, Kanupriya Agarwal, who was born just sixty-seven days after Louise, claimed as an IVF success by Dr Subhas Mukherjee, but whose birth took until 2008 to be credited to him. Until then he was pilloried, with some international disbelief, and his passport taken away, possibly because the government did not approve of his work. This prevented him from attending collaborative meetings internationally, and tragically, in a foreshadowing of the controversy that was to dog IVF for years, he took his own life in 1981, with some still disputing the veracity of his claim.

This slow progress was despite the fact that scientists across the world were working around the clock to replicate Bob and Patrick's achievement.[2] Soon, however, there was a flurry of successes; 1981 saw the first IVF baby in the US, and in February 1982 there was one in France. This was followed in August that year by Israel's first IVF birth. The success rate was still extraordinarily low, however, and given that Bob and Patrick had experienced

---

2　　Kate Brian, 'The amazing story of IVF: 35 years and five million babies later', *The Guardian*, 12 July 2013, www.theguardian.com/society/2013/jul/12/story-ivf-five-million-babies

over 450 failures in the lead-up to Louise's birth, there were naturally doubts in my mind about how viable this technology was going to be. During my Cambridge research I'd carried out many successful embryo transfers in rodents, but it was another matter to do it in humans. With my mice I'd had the luxury of removing an egg or embryo from one animal and transferring it into another – after all, a mouse doesn't much mind whether her offspring come from her. But in human IVF our task was to take an egg while still in the follicle, fertilise it, develop it for a few days, and then transfer it back into the same woman (who was still recovering from the physical stress of having her egg removed in the first place). Despite this I knew an embryo was an embryo and never doubted it had the potential to work.

In those days at Bourn Hall we didn't know how to manipulate a woman's cycle to produce eggs on demand which meant we had to work to her natural, spontaneous cycle. This led to each woman having a ten-day stay in the clinic, with her urine being tested every two hours during the day and twice at night to detect when she would begin ovulating; this became known as the infamous 'wee run'. What's more, because the Louise Brown embryo had been transferred into her mother at night, Bob believed this was the best time for every subsequent transfer. This led to me working – literally sometimes – twenty-four hours a day. I'd married my wife Janet five years earlier and had just become a father myself, so I suppose you could say babies were keeping me up at night on both fronts.

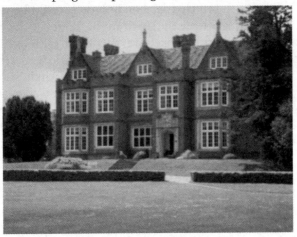

Figure 2.2: Bourn Hall Clinic

If you'd have visited Bourn Hall then, you'd have approached the main entrance without seeing the portacabins at first. There was also a barn area which was more attractive than the cabins and where my office and the endocrine lab were located. As you walked through the front door of the hall you'd have been greeted by a receptionist, after which you'd have continued to Patrick's office for a consultation on the right of the main entrance. It was a grand, bay-windowed room with a private examination area and en-suite bathroom. As for the scientific facilities, you wouldn't have believed the embryology lab if you were to see it today. Utterly unsophisticated, it was attached to one of the portacabins, with the culture medium being made by Jean in a little area round the back. Bob and I carried out the embryology in a poky room darkened by drapes over the only window because we were concerned about the effect of light on gametes and embryos. Patrick and John did the theatre work in the same portacabin, separated from us by a purpose-designed stable door. There was much creaking as we moved about. Our administration team and the endocrine lab staff handled the hormone testing, assisted by nurses who looked after everyone. Working in these close quarters imbued us with a spirit of pioneering camaraderie that stayed with us for the rest of our lives.

Our patients were accommodated six to a portacabin. As soon as the urine test flagged up the hormone surge indicating ovulation, Patrick or John would marshal a theatre team, I would be notified, and then either Bob or I would be there to collect the egg at any time of day or night. I felt for the women when we carried out this procedure. Patrick or John would have to infuse CO_2 into their abdominal cavity to do a laparoscopy, which gave the patients considerable pain in their shoulders as the gas dissipated afterwards. The main aim was to recover the egg as it matured in a tiny sac (called the follicle) within the ovary. They then aspirated the egg, together with its follicle fluid, into a little tube which they handed over to Bob or me in the lab through the top half of the stable door. Once we received the tube of yellow follicular fluid, we tipped it into a petri dish and tried to identify the egg by looking at it under a microscope. At that stage the egg, which was ten times smaller than a full stop, was surrounded by thousands of nursing cells. The whole thing looked like a microscopic cumulus cloud – it's called the cumulus mass. Our next task was to see if this mass contained an egg, which wasn't always the case. Once we'd inspected the fluid we had to rapidly communicate our findings to Patrick or John in the theatre, because if we hadn't found an egg they'd flush and aspirate the follicle again. This could occur many times before we finally obtained what we were looking for, and all the while the woman was lying there under general anaesthetic.

In the meanwhile we prepared the man's sperm before mixing it with the egg in a test tube. We learned the most important part of this was to clean it fully from the seminal fluid in which it was produced and therefore devised various methods of doing so. Each time we came up against a new problem with the sperm we had to find a way of safely removing the thousands of sperm needed to incubate with the egg, and sometimes the men didn't even have thousands of sperm, let alone the millions contained in the average ejaculate. Over time we found men could have many different sperm problems, including conditions we hadn't even known existed before.

We needed a minimum of 2,000 sperm to mix with the egg and its cumulus mass, which we did in a small test tube. The egg and sperm were gently mixed with a special combination of carbon dioxide and air, along with the ingredients in the test tube culture medium, to create the ideal incubating environment. On top of this test tube we placed a plastic lid, which we clicked into place to form a seal. This was put into a holding dish which was in turn placed into a large, bell-shaped glass jar called a desiccator. The role of the desiccator was to create a fail-safe environment for the eggs and sperm should the lid on the test tube accidentally come loose. A vital part of this task was to ensure the connection between the lid and base of the desiccator was well greased to create an airtight seal. We didn't have incubators so this desiccator had to act as one, and a special gas was manually flooded through a valve at the top. Finally the desiccator went into a warming cabinet which was maintained at 37° centigrade. It was a crude system, but it worked.

Within the first twenty minutes of placing the egg and sperm inside the desiccator, the heat in the warming box would cause the gas to expand which would make the top of the desiccator 'pop' from the seal holding it to the base. Because this was impossible to see, and given the pop came and went in a microsecond, it was easy to come in the next day to find the special air mixture had gone and the culture medium had turned alkaline. This stopped the embryo dividing and undid all our hard work (and we only had one precious egg per cycle). To stop this happening I'd have to return to the desiccator after fifteen minutes to release the pressure using a special valve at the top, and again after half an hour to make sure. Sometimes I'd return home at midnight only to wake with a start at 3 am convinced I'd not released the pressure properly, so I'd return to the clinic just to hear that comforting 'pssst' as the valve released.

On the morning after the egg and the sperm had been mixed I'd check if the egg had been fertilised. This was an onerous task I'd always carry out holding my breath – in fact, sometimes I had to remind myself to take one. I separated the cells surrounding the delicate egg using a technique that was extremely crude by today's standards. Taking two injection needles, I'd gradually tease away the outside cells, working my way slowly towards the egg. Peering through the microscope, I could see the tiny ends of the sharp injection needles and look right into the centre of the egg. I can only describe this process as like using two axes to peel the skin off an orange without touching the pith. What's more, I had to do it at a precise time so I could decide if the egg was fertilised.

If I spotted two tiny circles inside the egg I knew one was the genetic 'packaging' (the chromosomes containing the genes) from the sperm in what's called the male pronucleus, and the other was the female pronucleus containing the woman's chromosomes. When the egg has these two pronuclei it's called a zygote: it's fertilised but the parental genetic material is still independently contained within it. These pronuclei arrive about eighteen hours after the sperm has fertilised the egg, and disappear before the egg splits into two cells. Before a fertilised egg starts dividing the pronuclei fuse and become invisible, combining to form the embryo's genetic material. In rare cases, two or more cells may form but no pronuclei; I knew if I saw this that the dividing cells wouldn't create a viable embryo. Alternatively two sperm may enter the egg, creating three pronuclei; this would produce an abnormal embryo that probably wouldn't implant, or if it did, would likely end in a miscarriage or an abnormal baby. You can see how imperative it was to inspect the cells for the pronuclei and check that fertilisation was progressing normally.

In those days we'd put the embryo back in the woman three days after we extracted her egg because that was the timescale that had worked for Louise Brown. Placing the embryo in the woman's uterus was a highly delicate operation. I'd draw up the almost invisible embryo into a catheter under a microscope, walk with it into the theatre, and hand it to either Patrick or John to insert it into the woman's uterus. They'd place the catheter in position and I'd depress the syringe gently to eject a tiny amount of fluid containing the embryo. Because Patrick believed gravity might increase the likelihood of embryos implanting successfully, the women were asked to kneel forward with their bottoms in the air while this was done – the so-called 'knee-chest position'. One day a young but eminent doctor visiting from the US witnessed Patrick and I carrying out such an embryo transfer and asked, 'Patrick – why is this lady in the knee-chest position?' Patrick's typically gruff response was, 'Boy, have you never heard of gravity?'

It turned out later that the effect of gravity on implantation was a myth, and it took Patrick some time to abandon that practice, but we were feeling our way with everything. For instance, we noticed as time went by there appeared to be a jet lag factor in the timing of ovulation for our American patients as opposed to our British ones. It was caused by the pineal gland (which reacts to light levels) and its relationship with the hypothalamus, which is the area of the brain that releases the hormones needed for ovulation. This caused a six to eight-hour time difference in ovulation. Once the women had been in the UK for a month or two, for instance for a second round of treatment, they'd move onto the UK sequence. This remarkable sign of the body's natural rhythms was one of the many areas we studied over the years.

After the embryo transfer, the woman would return to the ward for the rest of the night and I often wondered whether she got much sleep. Compared to today, it was extremely basic IVF. We'd simply mix sperms with eggs, place the resulting embryo into our patient, and keep our fingers crossed.

I learned something interesting during that time. The process of putting the embryo back into the woman is a critical part of IVF because obviously if it doesn't implant, the painstaking work beforehand is lost. John had an extraordinarily gentle way of doing this, which meant his success rate was disproportionately high compared to Patrick's. If all our transfers at Bourn Hall had been done by him I think, in retrospect, we'd have had a higher success rate than we did. In fact I recently asked John how many embryo transfers he'd carried out when he'd worked with Bob and Patrick in Oldham prior to Louise Brown's birth, and was astonished to hear it was none (he'd been an assistant to Patrick but hadn't been hands-on). I'd always wondered why it took Bob and Patrick ten years and over 450 failures before they had success, and now I may have the answer. Patrick took the standard approach to gynaecology at the time, which was quite aggressive and no doubt caused stress for the woman's body, whereas John carried out the transfers in an extremely slow, precise way. Even today it matters a lot who does the embryo transfer. So Bourn Hall relied incredibly heavily on John in those early days, especially when Bob and Patrick were travelling a lot.

Bob didn't want me to give up my research post at Cambridge so I remained lecturing and researching mammalian reproduction there while also working at Bourn Hall. It was a delicate juggling act. I'd typically get up in the morning, do the egg collection round at the hall, return to Cambridge for my teaching and research, then return to the hall to carry out fertilisations or check where embryos were in their growth cycle. Then I'd rush home to grab some dinner, coming back again at 10 pm to assist with the embryo transfers. If there was a woman who was about to ovulate I'd stay to do the egg collection, which meant my following day would be messed up because the time of day I extracted the egg had an impact on when I could mix it with the sperm. All my work depended on our patients' natural, spontaneous cycle, so I was constantly on standby.

Nor were these my only responsibilities. Because Bourn Hall was the only independent IVF clinic in the world in its early years, Bob and Patrick were in huge demand for speaking and lecturing internationally, leaving John and me to handle the cases day-to-day. Eventually Bob said to me, 'Look Simon, you've got to start doing some of these lectures', so we now alternated work at Bourn and giving international lectures. It was an intense time. Between working at the university, labouring day and night in the clinic, and travelling abroad to give lectures, I had little time for a personal life – I even had to give up my beloved sport. It wasn't as if we had the luxury of modern technology to help us, either. If you're over a certain age you'll remember what slides were and how labour intensive they were to produce – there was no PowerPoint in those days. I'd have to ask a secretary to type them out, and the photographic department to create the slide itself, a process that could take six weeks. This meant Bob and I only had one set between us for our numerous talks, which sometimes caused comical difficulties. On one occasion Bob and I agreed that to enable us to give back-to-back lectures in different countries, I'd finish off my cases at Bourn Hall and then dash to the arrivals hall at Heathrow to pick up the slide set from him. Unfortunately I was delayed by a difficult egg collection and set off too late. Frantically driving towards the airport, I spotted a 'meet and greet' parking sign on the other side of the dual carriageway. Swinging the car around like a madman, I bumped over the central reservation barrier and headed straight for the drop-off zone. 'Take me to the terminal, please!' I begged one of the drivers. Fortunately the chap was free so I tossed him my keys and he drove my car to arrivals. As I rushed into the hall I spotted Bob's back retreating; he'd obviously assumed I wasn't coming and given up. 'Bob!' I yelled. 'Come back!' The following scene was like something out of a movie, as we zig zagged towards each other like separated lovers with only a second to say goodbye. Bob thrust the slide carousel into my hands and I gave him a two second update on the egg collection at Bourn, then careered off to catch my flight. Which I did – just about. Little did I appreciate this kind of frenetic lifestyle was to be my lot for some time, in fact for most of my professional life.

***

Between 1981 and 1985 the team at Bourn Hall grew exponentially. By 1982 Bob wasn't doing much lab work as he was travelling so much, so more doctors and embryologists were brought in. I was doing less too because my research at Cambridge took up so much of my time, but I was still very much involved. Throughout this I found working with John to be fabulous. He's the best patient-orientated doctor I know, and I'm glad to say he remains a close friend. At the hall we carried out hundreds of embryo transfers together. In fact, one of our earliest was for Louise Brown's mother, Lesley. Bob and Patrick were away at the time, so it was up to John and me to undertake the responsibility of giving the Browns their second child. Talk about pressure – I still remember that embryo transfer as if it was yesterday. Happily it resulted in the birth of Natalie,

Louise's sister, who later became the first woman conceived through IVF to have her own children naturally. Maybe that makes John and me the first IVF surrogate 'grandparents'!

The atmosphere among our patients was one of hope against all odds. There was no such thing as a 'success rate'; these women were simply there for the opportunity to conceive, however remote. For most of them the team spirit helped them to cope – we were all in the trenches together, both staff and patients. Everyone was involved in this unique experience, sometimes forming lifelong friendships. We ate in the dining room together where I met a huge array of people from the UK and all around the world. There were folk from every walk of life, even wealthy Arabs and gypsies, all united by the burden of infertility. It cost £2,000–£3,000 for treatment – the average annual income at the time was around £6,000 – which inevitably led to a preponderance of people with means. We had a sheikh from the Middle East who would have his wife's halal food delivered by Rolls Royce from Fortum & Mason twice a day, and another sheikh whose minder would hand out £50 notes to anyone who opened the door for him (which pleased the staff no end). One day this particular minder asked John the time, to which he replied he hadn't got a watch. The next thing John knew, up popped the minder with a magnificent, diamond-studded, white-gold watch by Omega; I think John had it valued for about £6,000. I did try dropping hints that I'd be saved my regular walk up the hill if I had a car, but to no avail. Mixed with these wealthy types, though, were many ordinary people who'd mortgaged everything they had for the chance of a baby. It was humbling to see them staying in the same place as royalty – all hoping and praying for the same result. Many of these women hadn't told their friends and family they were having IVF because there was such a stigma attached to it, which strengthened the bonding even more.

It was our failures as much as our successes that drove us to keep improving our treatments. Sometimes, for instance, we weren't even able to harvest a single egg. This is almost unheard of today because we can extract eggs from several follicles at once, but without using drugs to stimulate follicle production we were limited to one egg from one follicle. We'd flush and flush and flush in an attempt to get it out, but occasionally to no avail. What's more, there were times when we'd mix the sperm and egg together and they didn't fertilise, despite the sperm appearing normal – why would that be? There were so many things we didn't understand. When we had those failures I was painfully aware that here was a couple who'd come to us to get pregnant, or at least have one embryo put back in the chance it would implant, and their hopes were dashed before they'd even started. On the occasions when an egg didn't fertilise I'd sometimes be approached quietly by the woman who'd ask, 'Is it my fault?' If I replied that it was probably an issue with the sperm, I'd occasionally get the response, 'In that case, please don't tell my husband.' I could only imagine what was going through her mind: a desire to protect him from shame, or an intention to find her own way to a baby without his knowledge?

Although it was an incredibly challenging and exciting time it was tough being pioneers when we had little to compare our work with, so in 1981 Bob asked me to help him organise the world's first IVF conference. The major players of the world's IVF community – a full twenty-five people at the time, most of whom have remained lifelong colleagues – flew in and it was a fantastic event. Bob picked them up from the train station one by one in his ancient Mini, which contrary to its usual performance managed not to break down. The conference itself was fairly chaotic because we were hardly experienced event organisers, but due to its being the first of its kind it carried enormous kudos. Even now I'm often asked for copies of the slides we showed, because it was so historically significant and helped start the spread of IVF expertise around the world.

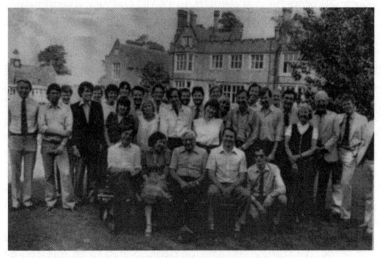

Figure 2.3: Bourn Hall world first IVF conference 1981

The conference also produced the book *Human Conception In Vitro*. The content for each chapter was generated by taped discussions from the event, which Bob and I listened to night after night in his little flat on the top floor of Bourn Hall. We read the transcriptions our secretaries had produced, wrote them up into chapters, put the relevant experts' names by them, and sent them out for approval. After a marathon writing session Bob poured me one of his favourite whisky macs and said, 'Look Simon, do you mind, I know you're doing a lot of work on this book but I've not had a chance to credit Jean Purdy much over the years. Is it ok if Jeannie's name goes on the cover alongside ours?'

'Of course', I replied. 'Why would I mind, given she's worked with you all these years?'

Imagine my surprise, then, when the book was published with only Robert Edwards and Jean Purdy credited as the authors – I was completely excluded. It was disappointing because of how much I'd put into it, but I swallowed it as the inevitable result of being the junior partner in Bob's venture. 'Tough luck, Simon', I thought – that's all. If I'd known then that we were to hold another conference in 1985 (popularly called the 'Second Bourn Hall Meeting'), which also resulted in a book – *Implantation of the Human Embryo* – and that the same thing would happen with this one, I might not have felt so sanguine.

The conference also marked a shift from Bob attempting to keep his work relatively secret and away from the prying eyes of potential competitors and critics, to a more collaborative approach. You have to remember how highly controversial our work still was, which made him wary. To put this antagonism against IVF into perspective, there was no way I could have studied it in humans at Cambridge – that could only happen at Bourn Hall. One day Bob issued nine writs for libel, including to the media and the Chairman of the British Medical Association (BMA), just to protect his name and our work. I'll never forget one evening when I was working late in a portacabin, finishing off a case. The door opened and in he stumbled, ashen faced. 'I've had a bad time with the lawyers from the BMA', he said. When I asked him what was wrong he explained his writ had resulted in the organisation pursuing a case against him, and pages had been found torn from his original research notebooks, a fact he couldn't explain.

It wasn't as if we were gung-ho about the social impact of our work. We stipulated that our patients had to be referred by a medical practitioner and also be married before we treated them. The referral rule was generated by Patrick to ensure we only received enquiries from patients who had some chance of success. I think the rule about being married was because our work was radical enough to be criticised as it was, without making it even more socially transgressive by treating single women. Times have changed now, of course; a few years ago there was a case in which a single, gay man had a child delivered by his mother who was acting as a surrogate for his egg donor.

There were also doctors who opposed us, for example Robert Winston (a tubal surgeon at the time) and Ian Craft (a competitor IVF pioneer). It was rather unpleasant. Craft had asked me to work for him a couple of times during 1980 and my refusal hadn't endeared me to him. Winston, who was always more embracing of the media than Bob and Patrick, was aggressive in his objections to IVF and denounced the validity of our work. So although Bob's international position was prestigious, locally there was hostility; as the saying goes, you're never a hero in your own land. This was reflected in the fact that Patrick never received the knighthood he set his heart on before he died, and although Bob was knighted, it took a long time. On more than one occasion, while we were scrubbing up for a case in theatre after the New Year's Honours List had been published, Patrick would mutter 'they've missed me out again'. Of course, in the end not only was Bob knighted but he also won the Nobel Prize for Physiology or Medicine; sadly as Patrick had died by then he couldn't join Bob in this great honour.

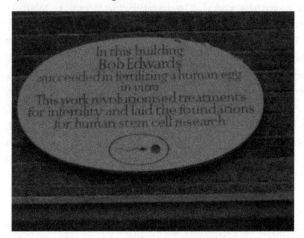

Figure 2.4: Plaque on the wall of the Physiology department at Cambridge University

Research-wise it was an incredibly active time for us. I published thirty articles with Bob during the five years I was at Bourn Hall, and during 1985 alone we managed fifteen between us.[3] What drove me to keep researching was the terrible feeling I'd have when I couldn't give a couple the baby they dreamed of, and – even worse – when I had no answers as to why I'd failed. However, the good thing was we were able to keep rapidly improving our techniques because we weren't hampered by the need to provide advance evidence of efficacy. We had an independent ethics committee to oversee our work but doing specific trials wasn't a pre-requisite for trying something new. If a patient asked for a different approach we could try it. Through this we learned, for instance, that if we occasionally managed to harvest two eggs instead of one and put two embryos back in the woman, we'd have a better chance of achieving a pregnancy. The Australians were having success with stimulating ovaries to produce more eggs, followed by the Americans and the French. So we started to carry out mild stimulation, and every time we returned two or three embryos we'd increase our success rate. Even then our live birth rate was only around 15 per cent, despite not dealing with the complicated cases we see today. As a comparison, in the UK's top IVF clinics we can now achieve a 35 per cent live birth from all ages of mothers, and over 50 per cent if the woman is under thirty-six.

Recently I gave a talk about the history of IVF at a symposium at the Royal Society of Medicine and a senior member of the HFEA was on the panel. They weren't impressed: 'Well, that was then and this is now, Simon. We can't allow progress unless we can be sure it works.' I come across this attitude all the time, but if we'd laboured under that system at Bourn Hall we'd never have been able to develop anything better, and nor would others elsewhere.

It was inevitable that the concerns about IVF felt by many would evolve into a formal investigation. Dame Mary Warnock started her commission into IVF during my time at Bourn Hall, and this would later become the Warnock Report.[4] In doing so, she asked representatives of various social groups to submit their thoughts. Lord Jakobovits, who was the Chief Rabbi of

---

3   See Author Cited Publications at the end of the book.
4   Mary Warnock, Report of the Committee of Inquiry into Human Fertilisation and Embryology. London: Department of Health and Social Security. 1984.

the UK at the time and an eminent medical ethics authority, came to visit. He had many questions to ask of me both as a Jew myself and as an IVF expert, and the outcome of this would later be distilled into Orthodox Jewry's submission to the Warnock Commission. Various elements of IVF troubled him, such as the freezing of embryos. 'Because I lived through the Nazi era', he said, 'the potential for damage to the embryo deeply affects my thoughts, even though I can see there's good intention behind the process. To me, embryos in a deep freeze each have the potential to become a human being. I have an enormous problem with them sitting there and, if in the wrong environment, being abused. But I don't have a religious reason to be against it.' We had many fascinating debates about this and other aspects of cutting-edge science.

We also discussed the topic of cloning. My work with animal embryology had taught me that splitting a single embryo into two was not only possible but effective in improving success rates, and I genuinely hoped I could significantly increase the number of pregnancies we achieved if I had more than one embryo to work with from each woman. So I started doing this with human embryos too, just to see what would happen. In a sense I was creating a natural clone by twinning the embryo, although I'd never have had the confidence to transfer them. I asked Lord Jakobovits: 'Why is that unacceptable? Nature does it when identical twins are created, so why can't we do it if we're increasing our patients' chances of them becoming pregnant?' Not that I approve of actual cloning (rather than the twinning approach) – so far, it's medically unsafe and as such must remain outlawed. However, our ethics at that time came from a combination of what we thought was right and what the patient would accept. No guidelines or regulations had been established.

In 1983 I was invited to Canada as the Pfizer Travelling Fellow to debate ethics with politicians who were deliberating on IVF. I was only thirty, and soon learned it was one thing being master of my scientific subject, but quite another to discuss this hugely contentious field with national politicians. The experience did, however, give me the confidence to expand my remit to more than just science, and stood me in good stead for standing up for my beliefs in future. As a way of exploring this, I wrote a paper called 'Cognitive Dissonance and the

Argument of Potentiality',[5] in which I asked whether what was under a microscope was a potential human being or a human being with potential. Or was it just a ball of cells that wasn't yet defined as anything, given most early stage embryos don't develop into viable embryos in any case? Without doubt the religious world saw these clumps of cells as either persons or potential persons, but what if I were to split a four-cell embryo into four separate cells and grow them into four full embryos? Would I then have identical quads, and if they didn't survive would that be homicide? And if so, of how many people – one or four? I spent many hours debating this in my head because I wanted to be sure I wasn't doing anything wrong. I knew our work was out of step with many people's views – for example, those of the *Times* cartoonist who drew a picture of a baby in a test tube with a pair of scissors cutting off its arm – but I also had the view that if people genuinely believed life began at conception, and if – as we know happens – an embryo can die naturally before it grows into a baby, why didn't we give it a conception certificate and a name? Or even a funeral? IVF was throwing up many new conundrums.

The upshot was that although I was troubled by the negative opinions of others, I never had doubts about the ethics of creating embryos that might not survive, because 60 per cent of them would never go on to become babies in a natural environment. There were also (and still are) conflicting views between religions about when life starts. Jewish law, for instance, doesn't give viability to a foetus until forty days, whereas for Catholics a human being is created at conception. To me, what I had under a microscope possessed a certain moral status because it was a couple's chance of a child. But I combined that with knowing it wasn't sentient. Being a clump of cells which may or may not develop to become a placenta or even a foetus, it was as much a 'person' as the cells that come from my gums when I brush my teeth. That's not to say the life I see in a cell isn't remarkable, but I don't think life begins at the moment of fertilisation. As for manipulating an embryo, this was certainly not the same as chopping off an ear, for instance. It was simply doing something to some cells that were the product of conception. People might say, 'How do you know it

---

5   Fishel 1988.

wasn't an Einstein you just killed?' My answer would be: I know, because it wasn't. As a clinic we went through years of work in IVF respecting the views of abolitionists and absolutists, but we didn't give up just because we faced opposition.

There was one horrifying time in 1984 when the prevailing hostility towards IVF threatened to land me in jail. I'd published a paper with Bob in the journal *Science*, explaining how Bob and I had discovered the human embryo is the source of a substance called hCG (the hormone now detected by pregnancy tests) and measured the timeline of its secretion.[6] I'd taken and analysed tiny amounts of culture medium from around an embryo in a dish, which included 'spare' embryonic cells that weren't part of the embryo itself. This process told us the hormone came from the very early placental tissue that was developing from the fertilised egg. After the paper was published we were both served with writs for murder. In fact the 'oldest' embryo we'd worked on was thirteen days post-fertilisation before it demised, and didn't show signs of developing early embryonic cells, only what we call trophoblastic tissue (the precursor to placental tissue). This meant it wasn't technically an embryo. What's more we had not touched the growing cells, only observed them. Still, it was enough in the minds of some to believe we'd committed murder. I was consumed with worry until eventually the Department of Public Prosecutions informed us there was no case to answer.

You can see what a rollercoaster ride my five years at Bourn Hall was, and by 1984, unbeknownst to me, they were starting to come to an end. Around this time, the atmosphere at the hall became somewhat tense and depressing. Jean would often come into my office to confide in me tearfully about her deteriorating working relationship with Bob. On one occasion she'd been due to go on holiday to Egypt and he wouldn't let her go, saying he needed her around. Tragically she died at the age of thirty-nine from a melanoma. She had a strange relationship with Bob and I had the impression he felt terrible about the way it ended.

Another frustration for me was Bob's lack of vision for Bourn Hall as a franchise. I knew many wealthy backers wanted to open IVF units and that there would be funding available for us to expand. 'Bob, this is our opportunity', I'd say. 'We could

---

6   Fishel Edwards et al. 1984a.

bring money into the hall if we opened more clinics. Not only would more people benefit from IVF but it could become a beacon of research and development. We could even ally it to Cambridge University – imagine the merger of those two great brands. Let's at least investigate it.'

But Bob had no truck with the idea. 'Simon, do you want to be constantly on a plane flying from one clinic to the next, or do you want to be doing the work you love?' (the irony was, we were on a plane to a teaching assignment at the time).

Eventually I went to see Alan Dexter, the Financial Director of Bourn Hall. He was the person who'd put together the original financial deal which made the place happen, and he agreed with me. But in his genial way he told me that if I wanted to make those changes, I'd have to do my own thing. I was surprised at how frank he was but he certainly planted a seed in my mind. I'd never considered going it alone before.

So why did I eventually resign? The trigger was a visit from a man called Peter Jackson, a Zimbabwean junior embryologist working in Cape Town, South Africa. He'd asked me and Bob if he could visit us to learn about our work. This wasn't unusual as we regularly welcomed visitors from around the world who were keen to discover what we were doing, including several gynaecologists from South Africa, and we'd happily show them around. Bob agreed instantly to his visit, which took place while I was on annual leave. While I was away I received a call to say he'd arrived, and I confirmed it was all arranged and that he should be welcomed in. To my surprise two of our senior staff members responded that they didn't want him in the lab. 'That can't be right', I said. 'He's come all the way from South Africa on limited funds and in good faith.' They told me he could return to the pub where he was staying and then go home. I contacted Bob who – against his earlier agreement – asserted that unless Peter was a 'freedom fighter' against apartheid he wouldn't be allowed into the clinic (this had certainly not been the case with previous South African visitors). After much discussion he conceded that when I was back from holiday I could allow him to watch my work, but not when anyone else was around. I felt so sorry for Peter, and so hurt by Bob's stance, that I cancelled my leave and returned to Bourn Hall at once.

When the visit was over I sat down with Bob. 'I've been thinking about this. I don't work for those other staff, I work for you, and you're the boss. If you say a visitor can come in then he should come. Why should it only be when I'm on duty? I can't be here all the time. I had to cancel my holiday.'

'Well, that's just the way it is.' Bob replied. 'I have to consider my other staff.'

I was shocked by this and on the Friday of that week I handed Bob my letter of resignation. 'What's this?' he asked. 'I'm not having this.' He handed me back the unopened envelope. 'Just forget it.' In the end our compromise was I'd stay for a while before leaving; I didn't have another job to go to and it was clearly going to be easier for Bob if I made a slow exit.

Interestingly, I'd recently been invited to open the first IVF clinic in New York. I'd originally been hesitant in my response but now I'd resigned from Bourn Hall I felt free to follow it up. The clinic backers flew me there first class on Pan Am, where they informed me there was a consortium of doctors ready to start work. I was taken to a plot of land in the middle of Manhattan and told: 'This can be yours – build whatever you want.' In some ways it was like a dream come true because I had two young children and needed an income once I left the hall, but I had my doubts about it. What would it be like to re-locate my family to New York? My wife Janet flew over separately to look for houses and although she wasn't too keen on the move she accepted it given I was determined to go ahead. I turned to John, who'd become my confidante during our lunchtime running sessions around Bourn village, telling him I planned to make this move but that it would take a while to get it set up, and that I'd continue working at the hall in the meanwhile. Once Bob learned of my pending move to the US he seemed a little cool, but wished me luck with taking IVF to America.

While the New York clinic was in the planning stages and I was yet to leave Bourn Hall, John and I were invited to give a lecture on IVF to specialists from Nottingham University. Our invitees were previous visitors to the hall: Malcolm Symonds (Professor and Head of Obstetrics and Gynaecology at the university) and consultant gynaecologist Tony Tyack. Malcolm and Tony undertook private clinical work at the nearby Park Hospital in Nottingham, with Malcolm also holding an academic post at the university. One frosty November evening after a long day at the hall, John and I arrived to give our lecture in the hospital canteen. As my first slide came up I asked if they had a pointer. Tony said they certainly did. He strode over to a magnificent rubber plant – a Large Monstera – in the corner of the room, broke off the longest stem, trimmed it down, and gave it to me: 'Here, take this.' Something told me we were going to get along.

A few days after our lecture, John pulled me aside as we met for our lunchtime run and gave me some astonishing news. Malcolm and Tony wanted John and me to build an IVF unit at the Park Hospital in Nottingham. John had always been a bit of a trickster so I suspected he might be pulling my leg, but it turned out he was serious. 'John', I said. 'You know I'm going to New York. The guys are coming over next month with contracts – I'm going to do it.'

The reality, however, was that while I sounded confident about the US venture, I was feeling far from it. Exciting though Manhattan was, both my wife and I had doubts about bringing up our children there. We'd considered living outside the city but knowing how fluid my working hours were, I didn't relish the thought of a daily transit to and from Manhattan Island. The move would be more about the money and opportunity than our quality of life. Nottingham, on the other hand, was considerably nearer to Sheffield where Janet's family was based. Also, I was keen to work with John because we got on so well and I knew I could trust him – who knows what the American doctors would be like? As for John himself, he was desperate to leave Bourn Hall – he had his own ambitions and had risen as far as he could there. Eventually he won me over and I told the Americans I wasn't coming.

You can imagine how well this went down, and also envisage Bob's reaction when he heard that instead of going to America I'd be moving up the road to Nottingham with John to start a competitor clinic. His reaction was swift. He tried to cancel some overseas lectures I was due to give by telling the organisers, who were eminent people in my field, that I'd lost my credibility. Fortunately when the organisers told me about it they assured me they had no intention of cancelling and the talks went ahead as planned. The episode didn't bother me too much, I just felt it was a pity. I'd also agreed a book deal on the history of IVF called *IVF: Past, Present and Future*, which was to be edited by me and Bob. Bob had been delighted to land this project when I told him it was arranged, but as soon as he heard about my move to Nottingham he tried to get it stopped. When the publishers refused he withdrew from it and put pressure on Patrick not to write his chapter on 'Laparoscopy for IVF'; I knew this because I had a warm and friendly phone call from Patrick explaining he had no choice or pleasure in having to withdraw, and that he wished me well. Instead, John wrote that chapter and I invited Malcolm Symonds to be co-editor in place of Bob. It was published in 1986 and was quite a success; it was the first book about IVF to be translated into Japanese.[7]

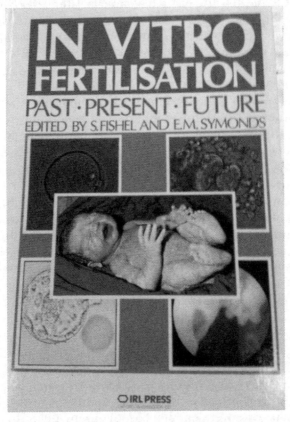

Figure 2.5: IVF: *Past, Present and Future* (1986)

After I left Bourn Hall, Bob and I had little contact for years. When I was eventually in legal trouble with my court case he phoned me up; surprised but pleased to hear from him, I asked if he would be a character witness at my forthcoming

---

7   IVF: Historical perspective. In Fishel and Symonds (eds) 1986.

trial. He replied, 'I'd like to, but this is something you've got to handle yourself.' In the end we had dinner together at Churchill College in Cambridge a few times before he died, and made our peace (or at least I did with him, I'm not sure if he ever did with me but it felt that way). In December 2009 I had lunch with him there, the year before he was awarded the Nobel Prize. Quietly he said to me, 'Simon, I think next year will be my year … but it's too fucking late.' I misunderstood, thinking he meant he was too old to care. Just a few months later I discovered he was slipping into vascular dementia. How terrible to think he must have known he had a chance of the honour but also that he wouldn't be capable of accepting it in a year's time. He died in 2013 and most people close to him believed he didn't fully know he'd received it; he certainly couldn't enjoy it.

It was only recently I learned that a while after I left Bourn Hall it was saved from bankruptcy by the drug company Serono (as it was then named). After this Bob left and founded the journal *Human Reproduction*, and after resigning from that project amidst various issues he founded another one. I felt it got a bit messy for him in the end. The irony is that the traits I admired most about him – his enormous resilience and the fact he never worried about what the establishment thought – were what made him most difficult to be with when we parted. I identified with him in many ways because what he believed was also what I believed: that if people don't want to support or accept the value of what you're doing, you have to keep ploughing your own furrow regardless. And in a way it helped me when I moved away from him, because once I'd made the break from Bourn Hall, I learned I was still in demand without him.

When I accepted the position at Nottingham it was decided I'd work in a similar way to the way I had worked at Bourn Hall and Cambridge, holding an academic research post at the University of Nottingham as a Reader, and as Scientific Director at our newly established IVF clinic at the Park Hospital. John was to work solely at the clinic; he was offered a university post but preferred to remain as Medical Director at the Park. Funnily enough Peter Jackson, the visiting embryologist from Zimbabwe, became my assistant there years later.

It's only now, when I look back on those extraordinary Bourn Hall days, that I realise what a unique era it was. We had the freedom and flexibility to change our treatments from one day to the next according to what our patients needed. We could form strong bonds with them too. And most of all it was just so exciting to go to work every day – for each and every one of us. Together we were laying the foundations for a medical treatment that was to change families around the world; it's no wonder that at IVF conferences now, delegates are often awestruck when they meet they meet one of the few remaining colleagues who worked at the beginning of Bourn Hall in any capacity. That alone is inspiring to me.

Chapter 3

Beginnings

1953–1980

But before we go on a journey eighty miles up the road to Nottingham, let's take a trip back in time to Liverpool. I was born into a traditional Jewish family there. My mother's parents were Ukrainian immigrants, hailing from what was then the USSR. So the story goes, they first met on their wedding day as Orthodox Jews did in those days, and their wedding present was a boat ticket to escape the pogroms in the USSR so they could begin a new life in the USA. Imagine two nervous seventeen-year-olds boarding a huge ship, knowing they would never see their families again. It docked at Liverpool on the way to America, but not realising they hadn't yet reached the land of the free, the newly married couple disembarked by mistake and found themselves with no choice but to settle in the land of rain instead. Liverpool in those days was smoke-laden, grimy, and poverty-stricken; as my mother used to say, 'If you didn't have a penny for the wick, you lived in the dark.' Although my grandparents didn't speak a word of English they had no choice but to make a life in their accidental home. My grandfather became a cabinet maker and my grandmother a housewife looking after their twelve children.

My mother Jane, their daughter, grew up in intense poverty and under the strict discipline of her parents. When she eventually met my father Joseph, a Jewish tailor, she told her mother she didn't want to marry him and whenever he visited she'd nip out the back door to avoid him. Eventually she was told she'd have to do the decent thing, because in her mother's view Joseph was a gentle chap and his father wore a gold tie pin. So she married him and had my sister Ruth, with me following on nine years later.

During my years growing up, neither of my parents were happy with each other, which didn't make for a harmonious household. My father laboured six days a week in his tailoring business and on Sunday he slept; in the winter Mum would wake him up for dinner and in the summer he'd garden, 'because it's the only place I have any peace'. This didn't matter much to me because I had a confidante in Ruth and loved being part of our wider family of uncles, aunts and cousins. They also came from poverty, with some of them managing to generate a huge amount of wealth before – for some of them – plunging back into destitution. Craftsmen and businessmen of various descriptions, with hardship giving them an aggressive desire to succeed, they were entrepreneurial. One example was the eldest in my extended family, Uncle Barney, who won a place at university but couldn't go due to lack of funds. His solution was to build a sizeable import-export business, becoming the first successful businessman in the clan. He changed his surname from Rosenblatt to Ross and called his company Benross, which is still around today.

Looking back, I was so naive and unworldly. Ruth, who became an apprentice hairdresser, would buy me Superman DC comics with her tips and I became a world authority on Superman. Most of my days were spent in my bedroom daydreaming with my comics; my career ambition was either to become an astronaut or a binman. When Ruth left home to marry Alan I was only nine, so suddenly there was an affection gap in my life. Luckily I carried on being close to both of them and eventually to their children too, babysitting for them as a teenager.

There was no education at home so everything I learned was from school. I have no memory of there being any books in our house, which was probably why I was such a painfully slow reader. Despite my naivety, or maybe because of it, I had a dogged perseverance about me. One weekend when on a camping trip in the Wirral for the Jewish Boys' Brigade, I fell out of line and was ordered to run up the local hill and not return until I'd touched the monument at the top. Four hours later, when I finally staggered back with clothes torn and soaking wet, I discovered the astonished leader had never actually expected me to do it.

Once I was old enough to walk myself to school my mum took herself off to become a nurse. Like many women of her day she had plenty of abilities and was an exceptionally energetic and determined person but didn't have the freedom to express herself career-wise. She also had the most magnificent singing voice, as did many in her family. In fact her brother Louis sang at one of the Liverpool theatres until his father found out and dragged him off the stage: 'Jewish boys don't appear in public.' My whole family led a fearful existence because my mother's parents had been outsiders and had taught her to keep herself to herself. One of her most memorable instructions to me was, 'Always keep your counsel – your good name is everything.' You can decide for yourself whether or not I kept this advice as I grew up.

At the age of eleven I graduated to the local senior school, The King David, which still exists today. I found myself sitting next to a boy called Jonathan Segal. He was holding an intriguing object with lots of writing and no pictures. 'Is that a book?' I asked incredulously. 'Yes, it's called Speed Six – it's about a green Bentley', he replied. 'Do you want to read it?' It was the first time I'd ever been given a book.

My education was hampered by the fact I didn't realise how short-sighted I was. I kept getting the wrong bus home, for which I'd be smacked for lateness. Eventually my mum had my eyes tested and from then on I could see the blackboard clearly. Despite that, I was a poor reader and never a good student; the constant refrain in my reports was 'could do better', and 'he should stop being a puppet to his peers' (what on earth did that mean?). But although I wasn't academic I never felt unpopular because I was sporty and somewhat mischievous, or lobbus as we would say in Yiddish. One evening my brother-in-law Alan, who'd become a substitute father to me by then, received a call from the local police station asking him to pick me up. I'd been nabbed for stealing hub caps and was suspected to be under the influence of cider. To my everlasting gratitude Alan sorted me out with a clip around the ear and promised not to tell my dad.

Things came to a head when the headmaster, Mr Beeby, told my mother I was in line to fail my O levels and that I'd better prepare myself to become a tailor like my father. I was devastated at this because I'd witnessed his daily grind all my childhood. Alan stepped into the breach, persuading Mr Beeby I was simply the joker in the pack and that I deserved a second chance; this spurred me into action on the academic front. For the first time I concentrated in class, did my homework, and studied for my exams, scraping five O levels and being accepted into the sixth form. Although I was informed I wasn't bright enough to take the three A levels needed for university, I was made Head Boy as well as House and Sports Captain – I may not have been a hard worker but I excelled at sports and found it easy to get on with people. As Head Boy I represented the school in all sorts of things. At our Speech Day in my final year, which was held at the Royal Liverpool Philharmonic Hall, I had to look after our guest of honour, the world-famous violinist Yehudi Menuhin. Listening to our school orchestra must have been one of the most tortuous experiences of his life, so appalling were we. After the performance I could see him struggling for words, finally coming out with: 'Keep practising – it's good to practise.'

Because I wasn't allowed to study for three A levels, university wasn't an option for me. I had no idea what to do with my life and toyed with many ideas. One of them was to do something medical, so I arranged to look around Alder Hey Children's Hospital. Two things hit me immediately: the number of children with horrific burns from the previous evening's Bonfire Night, and the horrible conditions that some of the children had been born with. There were some kids with no brains and others with huge heads due to water on the brain; this was relatively common then due to the lack of ultrasound scans in pregnancy. Shortly after that, I picked up my mum from her job as a psychiatric nurse to find she and her colleague had been badly beaten by a patient and her parent. This, together with my experience at Alder Hey, convinced me the medical profession wasn't for me. When I scraped two A levels in biology and chemistry (both grade Es – they were as bad as you could get) I was disappointed but not surprised. It was isolating, though. I knew I wanted to do something with my mind rather than my hands, but what?

One thing was for sure, I wasn't going into tailoring because I knew I was destined to achieve something different with my

life. Instead I took a year out, during which I went to night
school to study for a maths O level and an extra A level, in the
hope of getting into university. I achieved this while working
as a teacher's aide in a primary school in Speke, a tough area
of Liverpool. This turned out to be one of the most formative
experiences of my life. There was one family, the Kellys, who
had a kid in every year of the school; the dad was reputedly
always drunk and the much larger mother always seemingly
pregnant. I became attached to one of their children, Derek,
who would come to school without shoes on, and I gave him
extra support. When one of the teachers went on long-term
sick leave I ended up with a class of my own for six months as
well as helping other classes, but instead of finding it stressful I
thrived on the challenge. For the first time in my life I had a bit
of money coming in and bought my mum a washing machine,
because I couldn't bear to see her laundering our clothes in the
bath any longer. My regular treat was to visit the sauna at the
Adelphi Hotel with a teacher friend, as it was near my night
school. Once I went there on my own and found myself sitting
next to another naked chap, the comedian Tommy Cooper. He
looked 'just like that'.

After I'd gained my full complement of qualifications, I
applied to various universities and was finally accepted by the
University of Salford to study biochemistry and physiology.
This was marvellous given my poor A level results. Even in those
days I had the travel bug, and with the money I'd saved from
my year's teaching I went on several foreign adventures. These
included a trip to Scandinavia in Mum's old Triumph Herald,
a hitchhiking journey to Greece and Israel, and a Greyhound
bus tour around the US during which I almost got arrested for
working illegally at a gas station.

When I returned home it was off to Salford for me, where I
had some rum characters for lecturers. One of them was Emrys
Thomas, an Oxford-trained biochemist. On one occasion he
walked into the lecture hall, sat down, and then paced back
and forth in front of the large blackboard for a few minutes
while rubbing his chin. After a short time he announced in
his strong Welsh accent, 'I'm told I have to give you a lecture
on biochemistry. I know fuck all about biochemistry.' He
scribbled the names of five great biochemists on the board.
'Read them', he said. 'They know about biochemistry.' And out
he went.

At the end of term I sat an assessment exam, which true to my track record, I failed. My tutor, Dave Power, took me aside: 'If you repeat that result again you're out, and I think you'll find your ambitions to do anything academic are over. That's the tough bit. Here's the better news: you're not daft, and if you work and get a good degree, anywhere will have you and you can do what you like.' Somehow he made me realise it was time to grow up. So despite the fact that my joy in life was to play for the various university sports teams, I knuckled down and worked – and blossomed, thanks partly to a great teacher I'll never forget, Professor Orville-Thomas. At the end of the year I achieved a grade A in my organic chemistry exam which felt unbelievable – I'd never had an A for anything before. This encouraged me to throw myself into everything else, and by the end of my second year I felt like a proper student. When it came to finals results day in June 1974, I stood in front of the list of names and results on the departmental noticeboard and automatically cast my eyes towards the bottom. No 'Fishel, Simon' there. Gradually I moved upwards with a thudding heart until, with utter disbelief, I saw my name at the top, amongst only three to achieve a double first. Finally I'd proved I could learn.

After the excitement of my results had died down, I found myself pondering what to do with my degree and realised I would love to learn about virology. My tutor advised me to apply to Cambridge for a post-graduate position. 'You've got a first class honours from Salford', he said. 'Okay, you're thinking "it's only Salford", but it's a university, which means you can do whatever you like. Apply.' So I did, and took the night bus down to an interview. Amazingly I was accepted to do a virology PhD in the department of biochemistry.

Cambridge, my god! Once I started there my first impression was of how ridiculously old the place was; in my research office I had a wooden milking stool to sit on and an ancient bench to write at. For the first few weeks at my college, Churchill, I did nothing but absorb the people and I soon realised some of them were only there because they came from privileged backgrounds – they were well educated rather than brilliant. It wasn't long before I was handed a hair-raising challenge, which was to give a talk to the senior staff of biochemistry. This sounded daunting enough, but nothing prepared me for walking into the room and scanning the audience. Before me sat an eminent mixture of Nobel laureates and living legends, some of whom had given their names to the biochemical reactions I'd learned about at Salford. One guy was hardly still alive, and yet there he was waiting for me to impress him. I delivered probably the most embarrassing talk I've ever given, and the only reason I got through it was because I was such a great improviser and bullshitter when it came to answering the questions.

It was now 1975 and I threw myself into college soccer, rowing and martial arts. It was the way I always was – seeing life as fun. I loved being at college and got on well with my tutors but was rapidly falling out of love with virology. I wondered what I'd ever found interesting about those invisible molecules – I mean, what where they? Deciding to reduce my PhD to a master's, which I'd almost completed in any case, I applied for jobs outside Cambridge. One of the positions I was offered was at Harvard Business School; another was at Unilever. Not feeling sure which to choose I had a chat with one of my college tutors, Kenneth McQuillan. He said he'd be happy to advise me and while giving me a lift back to college in his old sports Volvo, asked me how things were going. 'Well, after I've got my master's, I'm leaving', I replied.

'What do you mean, leaving? You can't do that. Let's think. Have you heard of Bob Edwards?' he said. 'He's over in the physiology department and is doing some interesting stuff with reproduction. He's always looking for bright students to work with. Why not pay him a visit?' I thought about all the interesting people I'd miss if I left Cambridge and reckoned it was worth a try.

The next day I made what turned out to be the pivotal decision of my life, which was to walk the fifty yards from one science building to another, up five dusty flights of stairs, and into the office of Dr Robert Edwards. As I edged through his doorway I saw an unremarkable looking man in his fifties sitting in a tiny office. Glancing up, he said, 'Why are you coming to see me?' I explained I'd been doing a virology master's for a year, that my degree was in biochemistry, and that I'd decided virology wasn't for me but that I'd still like to carry on in research. We had an interesting chat, during which he talked about embryology – a subject I knew little about – and finally used a phrase I'd never heard at the university until then: 'I'll see what I can do.' I left feeling he might have well as said, 'Don't call me, I'll call you.'

However, shortly afterwards he asked me to return and as we talked I learned what a down-to-earth Yorkshireman he was – far more normal than the average Cambridge professor. He had such a rapid way of talking with his Yorkshire lilt I sometimes found him hard to understand, and it took a while before I could stop nodding vacantly at every other sentence. Years later, when we'd eat in college together and he'd be asked, 'Would you like dessert, sir?' he'd reply, 'You mean pud?' He was straight-talking, had a warm smile, and everyone meant something to him regardless of where they came from; this made him a bit of a maverick at Cambridge. So my chat with him was easy and direct, but the outcome still unpromising: 'I'd still like you to do a PhD with me but I've got no funding.'

At this point I assumed it was all over and even made plans to depart Cambridge; I'd already submitted my master's thesis so there wasn't much more for me to do. Packing up my things, I left it until the last possible moment to let Bob know I was leaving; maybe there was a chance the funding situation had improved. When I phoned him I expected to hear the worst but he said, 'Listen, Simon, I've just heard from the department head there's some money available for you to do a PhD in mammalian embryology, so would you like to join me? I can't guarantee we'll receive all we need, but it's a start.' I was going to work for Bob Edwards. I wonder what would have happened if that funding had come a week later.

After that I spent night after night reading up on embryology and reproduction, so I could understand the words Bob had used in our initial conversation. It was unbelievably exciting to think I'd be working with such an interesting man – I couldn't wait. Once I started he said to me, 'I'm going to give you three pieces of information regarding your area of research. In your first year I'll give you all the help you need. In your second year you and I must be equals. In your third year you'll be the expert and I'll expect to come to you for information.' I reckoned I'd better throw myself into my research then. This wasn't hard because it seemed amazing to me that, from the clump of animal cells I could see at the end of my microscope, could grow a pup or a mouse. I learned all sorts of fascinating variations on how embryos form and implant differently in various species of mammal and was even the first to demonstrate that the embryo could respond to its environment, that the womb had its own specific signals, and that there is therefore cross-talk between the embryo and womb.

In the end my first year's 'supervision' never really happened because Bob was already commuting between Cambridge and a hospital in Oldham near Manchester, where he was engaged with Patrick Steptoe in trying to make IVF babies. Despite this we still managed to spend a lot of time together because on 12 October 1979 we were both elected Research Fellows of Churchill College, Bob as a senior and me a junior (this might be the only time when a student and his supervisor have been elected to a college fellowship on the same night). Not only was he my PhD supervisor, but we also dined together regularly at college. Shortly before then I'd also been awarded the Beit Memorial Fellowship, a prestigious prize of which four a year were bestowed on students from the Commonwealth. I was only allowed to keep the stipend that came with one award, so chose the Beit Fellowship and had the prestige of the Churchill Fellowship too.

Because my PhD research was based on mammalian embryo development and implantation, and Bob's work was on achieving human fertilisation, we had many conversations around these areas over the following couple of years. We became good friends although I'm not sure anyone was truly close to him; he was a funny mixture of warmth and openness at some times and secretiveness at others. I knew he was working hard to create what later became known as a 'test tube baby' in Oldham and that he was having multiple failures in doing so, but he didn't talk much about it because, I assumed, it was depressing to discuss a project that wasn't going well. There was also an unspoken worldwide race to be the first team to create an IVF baby and he didn't want much of it to come into the open. In addition to that there were many people who strongly disapproved of his work and didn't think it was wholesome or ethical, including two senior PhD students who later became eminent in their fields. They both eventually came around to it, though. One of them, Richard Gardner, went to Bourn Hall years later with his wife to have a baby through IVF (as he stated publicly), and the other, Martin Johnson, was to accept Bob's Nobel Prize on his behalf when Bob was too ill to travel to Stockholm.

Once Louise Brown was born in Oldham on 25 July 1978, Bob's world changed. My later colleague John Webster once told me that, as he and Patrick Steptoe were on their way to the operating theatre to deliver Louise Brown, Patrick said to John,

'This is going to be bigger than man's landing on the moon.' He was right. The Browns were besieged by the press for months and even years after baby Louise came home, and Bob achieved a kind of celebrity status along with them. This was less the case at Cambridge because there was still international concern his work was unethical or even duplicitous. Had he and Patrick achieved a world-first, or was it a hoax? This was one of the reasons they allowed TV cameras to film the birth, showing Patrick lifting up Lesley Brown's uterus to prove there were no fallopian tubes. It's hard for us now to conceive of how far-fetched Bob's work seemed at the time. Nobel Laureate James Watson, who discovered the structure of DNA with Francis Crick, was viciously against IVF. He said, 'All you're going to get are teratogens – monsters.' He was joined by the Chairman of the British Medical Association who denounced it as unethical, and there was a famous quote I've never forgotten from one newspaper: 'The work of Steptoe and Edwards is worse than a backstreet abortionist in Bangor.'

Three months after Louise's birth, Patrick had to retire from the NHS due to his age and this led to the closure of the IVF facility at Oldham. It took two years for him and Bob to decide what to do next, but in 1980 they created the world's first private IVF clinic at Bourn Hall. Until it opened, Bob worried the place would never get off the ground, as their US backers had withdrawn due to concerns about litigation in the event of abnormal births. Eventually the pair gained alternative funding to open the clinic and asked me to join them as Deputy Scientific Director. I had no hesitation in accepting and became part of the founding team.

I remember walking up to Bob's office in the physiology department shortly before the clinic was to open and getting as far as the third flight of stairs, when a senior member of the department stopped me. He knew I was to join Bob there and said, 'Fishel, I've been wanting to have a word with you. I need to give you some advice. Do not give up what could be a brilliant research career to work with the devil'. This shook me. I wasn't sure if he meant Bob or the work he was doing, but I'd never seen him as the devil, and still believed that because we knew IVF could work in animals (and it clearly worked in Lesley and John Brown's case), it could also be successful in humans.

So that's how it all started – and how my life changed irrevocably. You might wonder why I was so eager to join a venture that had, at that point, produced multiple failures, only two successes (another baby had been born shortly after Louise), and attracted worldwide condemnation. There were two factors that drove me. First, from the moment I started working with Bob, I was fascinated by the science of reproduction. I was captivated by the eggs and the sperm and how they combined to become an embryo – these were things I could see, feel, and understand. The magic of witnessing a new life form in front of my eyes with the fertilised egg dividing into cells – how the hell do they know what to do? – was indescribable. That single egg along with its sperm, nine months later, would become at least fifteen trillion cells organised into tissues, organs, a nervous system, and an amazing human brain. Secondly I revelled in becoming knowledgeable and beginning to feel, for the first time in my life, as if I was on an intellectual par with other academics. I couldn't get enough of it.

I was also moved by the idea of giving parents the chance of a child and a family. Although I was yet to experience the full emotional impact of this, it was a thrilling prospect. And I had a stubbornness about me that meant I wasn't put off by all the well-respected people who disagreed with it. I believed in Bob, who had an encyclopaedic knowledge about reproduction and who searched everywhere for ways to keep doing what he believed in. And I believed in myself. I decided if IVF didn't work I'd go down with the ship, but in the meanwhile I'd enjoy the voyage. Bob's secretary, Barbara Rankin, could see how important my support was to him, and his to me. One day she took me aside. 'Simon, just let me give you a word of advice. Never leave Bob. That's all I'm going to say.' I didn't understand why she gave me this warning at the time, but five years later her words were to return to haunt me.

Bourn Hall was poised to open and we knew nothing was guaranteed. Would we be able to create further babies? What would happen if any of them had abnormalities? And what if Watson was right? In early 1980s there was no way IVF was proven in anyone's mind – it still had a long way to go.

Chapter 4

Nottingham to Rome and Back

1985–1991

Although my years at Bourn Hall had drawn to a close, the world of IVF was expanding rapidly, attracting the attention of funding backers with deep pockets who'd seen the growing demand from infertile couples. This wasn't lost on me and led to what I fondly call my 'Bill Gates moment'. As the story goes, Bill Gates once approached IBM to explain what he was doing with this thing called Windows and to ask if it would be interested in the software.

'Personal computers?' IBM said. 'Nobody will want them.'

It had been the same for me when I'd suggested to Bob that we expand the Bourn Hall franchise, and now again when I approached managers at the private Park Hospital in Nottingham with my idea to set up a group of IVF clinics rather than just the one at the Park. I could see the potential in IVF and described how it could transform people's lives. 'Well, it seems interesting', they said. 'But infertility treatment isn't exactly a crucial issue – we can't see it becoming big enough for that.'

But I'm getting ahead of myself. When I first started at Nottingham there was much work to be done to get the Park

IVF clinic up and running in the first place. If you remember, Tony Tyack was a consultant gynaecologist at the Park Hospital and Malcolm Symonds was Head of Obstetrics and Gynaecology at Nottingham University. Together they'd asked me to fill a combined academic role at the university and a clinical one, alongside John Webster, at the IVF clinic at the Park.

The hospital was owned by a small consortium of doctors, including Tony. However, a private provider, American Medical International (AMI), was in the process of buying them out. This meant I ended up being closeted in a series of clandestine meetings at the Haycock Hotel on the A1 with John, a representative from the Park Hospital, the American head of AMI in the UK, and his corporate lawyer. These were followed by further discussions at AMI's head office at Cornwall Terrace in London, during which we hammered out a contract in which it was agreed John and I would run the Park's new IVF unit. In 1985 a deal was finally struck, and as it turned out that AMI – in the new guise of BMI – later became a partner in my current chain of IVF clinics, CARE Fertility. In these consultations I kept coming across a young lawyer from AMI, Stephen Collier, who I was later to discover would be pivotal to my future – for reasons I'm glad I didn't know at the time.

The combination of research and academia with clinical work meant everything to me because I wasn't interested in restricting myself to private IVF practice alone; research was a vital part of my mission to improve IVF treatments. While I'd been at Cambridge I'd felt massively frustrated that, due to the pariah status of IVF, the university couldn't be part of any pioneering work on it. Also, welcoming visitors from around the word at Bourn Hall had made me realise there was a desperate need to train practitioners. I knew the twin aspects of my academic work – the research and the training – would be impossible if I was working purely for commercial benefit at a private clinic. It had been my dream for years to create a beacon of research and practice, and if I couldn't do it at Cambridge, I thought, 'Well, I've got my own patch now. I'll do it in Nottingham.'

It was a hostile environment we were working in back then. In 1985 there was no guarantee IVF was ever going to be acceptable; it was only in 1990, when parliament finally gave it the thumbs-up, that it was publicly backed. In fact there was a worrying time before the vote when I thought it might go against us and close down IVF entirely. I have to give Robert Winston much of the credit for the vote going our way. He'd recently been one of the doctors at the Hammersmith Hospital in London who'd first screened out a genetic disease from an embryo, enabling a boy to be born without it. He used this, together with his media-friendly profile, to lead an almost single-handed campaign to push IVF through parliament. This was instrumental in overturning the negative opinion many MPs had about our work and prevented it from being banned in the UK.

So there I was, fighting for IVF and also for my dream to teach, train, and research as well as run a bloody good clinical IVF unit. And that's exactly what I ended up with. Nottingham University saw my work at the Park Hospital as an integral part of my research because I was continuing to evolve my work in human reproduction in ways that hadn't been done before. And the hospital saw my research at the university as an excellent opportunity to keep it ahead of the field. The future looked good, although I still had my own battles to keep my international connections alive after leaving Bourn Hall.

I knew to drive my research forward John and I had to achieve top results at the clinic, and we worked hard to build a reputation from scratch. Luckily the local doctors supported us; prior to our arrival the only help they'd been able to give infertile patients was to refer them to Malcolm who, with his team, would offer to stimulate ovulation or inject sperm into the woman's womb – this was called Intrauterine Insemination. Now both the doctors and Malcolm could send their patients to us and this, together with our early successes, meant the clinic quickly took off. I have to credit John with a large part of our excellent clinical results. His drive was different to mine as he was a purely patient-focused doctor, which meant he provided a stabilising counterbalance to me when I got excited about pushing forward the boundaries of research. And having someone who was calm and well-liked by patients, and who handled the process with professional ease, was fantastic.

Initially I carried out all the embryology myself and John was the only doctor; we had a secretary and a couple of nurses, but that was it. In those days as an embryologist my aim was to understand the science of infertility. I would examine absolutely everything we did, including what ovarian stimulation regimes we gave our patients and how the embryo was transferred. I was broad in my view of the field and published scientific papers covering a wide variety of topics, including one in the *British Medical Journal* which was the first to question whether IVF could influence the triggering of ovarian cancer.[8] When we first started up the clinic, however, there was only one method of IVF and it was basic. Much like we'd done at Bourn Hall, John would aspirate fluid from the follicles in the ovaries of our patients and I would search that fluid under the microscope to find eggs. I'd then take the sperm, free it from its seminal plasma, and make a judgement as to how far to concentrate it. Then I'd mix the sperm and eggs together, protecting them carefully in the right environment. The following day I'd see which eggs had been fertilised and exclude any that appeared abnormal, making sure the conditions were right for protecting the fertilising egg as it began its division into the few cells we call an embryo.

After two or three days I'd draw up the embryo carefully into a catheter and walk it to the adjacent theatre room where John was sitting waiting to receive it, and where the woman was lying on her back. More often than not her husband would be sitting by her side and they'd be holding hands. At that point John would take over and insert the catheter into her womb. Once he'd decided the catheter was in the right place he'd give me a nod and I'd gently (oh, so gently) depress the plunger on the syringe. This was a critical step because we didn't want to inject too much fluid, only just enough to expel the embryo. John would then remove the catheter extremely carefully so as not to drag out the tiny four to eight-celled embryo with it, and would hand it back to me to check under the microscope it had gone. It was like a well choreographed dance routine, except with a lot more holding of breath.

Once we were established at the Park Hospital, John and I realised we each needed a right-hand man, so John recruited his and I brought in Peter Jackson, the visitor to Bourn Hall from South Africa. Peter was a great learner and a loyal support, and his presence meant I could spend more time on my research while persuading the university to back me in developing more opportunities for IVF.

---

[8]   Fishel and Jackson 1989.

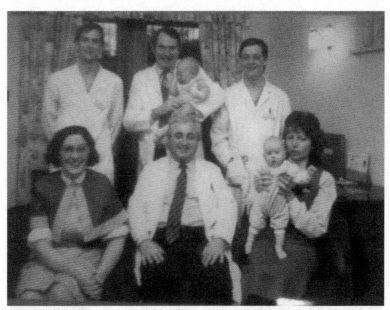

Figure 4.1: Early days at the Park. (*Top*) Me, John Webster, Peter Jackson (*Bottom left to right*) Sue Quickmire (Nurse Manager), Bahman Faratian (Assistant Medical Director), Heather Palmer (John's PA)

Our decision to take on more people proved to be a wise one when, in 1987, I was invited by the World Health Organisation to take IVF to China. I have to say, it's a testament to the support the Park Hospital gave me that they immediately said I could go. For me it was a huge honour to be the only clinical embryologist asked by the WHO to spearhead this, and along with three Swedish medical colleagues I spent six weeks teaching IVF to Chinese gynaecologists across four different cities. Over there they would only allow doctors to do the embryology, which was a challenge as these doctors had never seen any kind of embryo before. It was great fun and was crowned by the fact that we achieved the first Chinese IVF babies as a result.

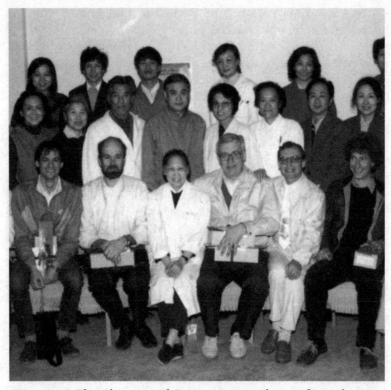

Figure 4.2: The Chinese and European team that performed some of the first IVF cycles in China in early 1987. **Bottom row from left:** Simon Fishel (UK), Matts Wikland (Sweden), Chau Billian (China), Karl Gustav Nygren (Sweden), Lars Marsk (Sweden)

I had some other interesting experiences too, for different reasons. In 1988, I appeared in an TV interview panel with MP Edwina Currie. She'd just been pilloried in the press for denouncing the majority of eggs in the UK as being infected with salmonella (cue a slurry of egg-related headlines). We were discussing IVF, and while I was making a point she interrupted me. 'Doctor, shut up for a moment', she said. Then she turned to the audience with a sly grin. 'Do you know, I've always wanted to say that to a doctor. It gave me such a good feeling.' This raised a titter and I replied, 'Edwina, the only problem you have with what I'm talking about is you just don't like eggs.' I like to think I got a bigger laugh; it was one of the only times I've been quick witted enough to get one over on a politician.

As time went by Peter and I were able to help many women to conceive and couples to become parents, but we still had to cope with the frustration of the failures we experienced. My main objective was to find ways of overcoming them, especially when eggs didn't fertilise. Sometimes we'd collect ten eggs and they would all remain unfertilised. Why? What could we do? We asked our patients if they would consider donor sperm but without using the embryo resulting from it; this taught us whether it was the egg or sperm that was causing the problem. We carried out many crossover studies like this because patients wanted answers, and over time we began to realise as yet unknown male sperm factors were a significant part of infertility. This was ground-breaking: until then infertility had been considered a purely female issue, but we showed there was more to it than that. In fact, today I'd estimate at least 40–50 per cent of infertility cases are caused by problems with the sperm.

In natural fertilisation the sperm has a cap on its head full of enzymes which digest the outer 'shell' of the egg and help it to penetrate inside – this results in fertilisation. But our studies showed us there were many occasions on which this failed to happen. We asked ourselves if there was a way for us to replace the enzyme action with an artificial 'shove' to help the process, which led me to experiment with pushing a sperm right up against the egg and then moving it across into the tiny area (the perivitelline space) between the inner egg and its outer shell (the zona pellucida). In effect this was sperm micro-injection, which I later called Sub-Zonal Insemination (SUZI). The fact I was able to combine my research position at the university and my clinical work at the hospital to develop this was an excellent example of the value of a joint commercial and academic enterprise, which was in many ways ahead of its time. I was then able to put a case to AMI and the hospital for the provision of funds to develop it, which they agreed to.

We knew SUZI worked experimentally but our next task was to figure out how the hell to do it in a practical way. An egg is ten times smaller than a full stop and a single sperm is twenty times smaller than that – how could we safely inject the sperm into the space between the egg's outer shell and its inner material? We needed equipment and it had to be small – microscopically small. Even if we could isolate the sperm and egg using some unknown set of tiny tools, how could we manipulate them under microscopic control? Ever resourceful,

Peter found a company in Cornwall run by a couple of charming chaps who'd come out of the electronics industry. My second wife Judy and I drove down in the snow to see them in my clapped-out Lada, which was always breaking down. This time it was the windscreen wipers and heating system that went, which meant Judy had to lean out of the window for five hours wiping off snow all the way while I drove as fast as I could.

When we finally arrived, bedraggled and hypothermic, we told them what we wanted to achieve. This was to hold the egg in place while it was in a petri dish in its culture medium, and then to use a glass needle to draw up the sperm; the needle would have to be twelve times thinner than a strand of human hair. So, we explained, we needed a tool to suck at the outer shell of the egg while holding it still, and another for the sperm. This one had to have a bevel at its tip, at a particularly precise angle, to approach the outer shell of the egg. This needle with the sperm, or glass pipette as it's known, would then have to get beyond the shell and up into the inner egg, which would mean it required an incredibly sharp tip to allow it to penetrate it. As if that wasn't enough we'd also need to place these tools under a specialised microscope, as the one we used for general IVF wasn't anywhere near powerful enough, and then be able to move them around with exquisitely fine control. And all with an accuracy in the region of a thousandth of a metre. Amazingly these engineers took on the challenge and designed the tools so we could make the pipettes ourselves.

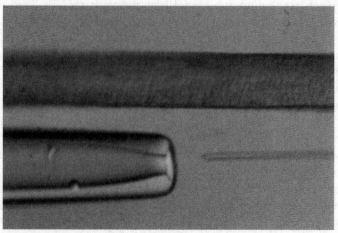

Figure 4.3: Needles for sperm injection with single strand of human hair above

Nowadays you can buy these pipettes off the shelf and eventually the company we visited developed into a substantial organisation called Research Instruments, serving IVF clinics worldwide. But back then we were only at research stage, with Peter and me using eggs that hadn't fertilised from patients who'd donated them and also carrying out some animal studies. Judy set up the equipment on our dining table at home; I'd call her up when I needed a particular number or variation of the minute pipettes and she'd create each one from scratch. Eventually we reached the point at which we could offer SUZI to real patients: desperate couples who had no-one else to turn to, their only other option being to use donor sperm.

There was, however, a stumbling block which I hadn't anticipated. While the Warnock Commission was working its way through its deliberations, two bodies had formed the Interim Licensing Authority, which had been set up by senior members of the Royal College of Obstetricians (RCOG), and the Medical Research Council. To my delight I was invited to London to talk to them about the growing field of IVF and looked forward to explaining the potential of SUZI. As I walked into the historic RCOG building on Regent's Park I could see a sumptuous lunch laid out on the boardroom table. 'This is great', I thought. 'We'll have plenty of time to talk about IVF over our meal.' However, just as I was about to enter the boardroom, one of the eminent obstetricians I was due to meet steered me in a different direction. I'd like to say it was to another room but it was just a corridor with a couple of chairs. It seemed the lunch wasn't for me after all.

As I leaned against the wall of the corridor facing this obstetrician, I was given some highly unwelcome news. 'We've looked at your research into SUZI and it's very interesting', he said. 'However, your task now is to prove it's safe before you use it on patients. No exceptions.'

Talk about a catch-22: how could I prove it was safe before I used it? The only time you can ever prove anything is safe is when you first put your toe in the water and try it for real. And it's a myth research will throw up all potential problems in any case. Thalidomide is a good example; it seemed safe after animal tests but in humans, look what it did in reality. I went away deflated because they'd set me a challenge I couldn't overcome: I had to use SUZI on human eggs and be able to transfer the resulting embryos to prove it worked, but I wasn't allowed to do that without knowing in advance it was safe. It's a paradox that dogged medical research then, and still does.

I was out of options for a while, but this was about to change. In 1987 I flew out to a conference in Florence, which was memorable for several reasons which still make me smile to this day. The first was that I took my mum along with me; she'd always wanted to see the city and it felt wonderful to treat her to a foreign trip. The airline lost my luggage and because it wouldn't have looked too impressive to give the plenary talk in my jeans and t-shirt, I had to go clothes shopping with her in the torrential rain. She was horrified at the prices for suits, as was I, although I consoled myself with the fact I was in the land of fashion so couldn't go too far wrong.

These experiences were special but what happened next was pivotal. After I'd given my talk, a squat, moustached man approached me, flanked by two much taller colleagues. The small man introduced himself as Severino Antinori and proceeded to bubble effervescently about how much he admired my work. Ebullient and full of enthusiasm, he was like a caricature of Italian exuberance. 'I want to work with you and I want you to work with me', he said, grabbing my arm. I felt a little taken aback but humoured him because he seemed interesting and had a cavalier twinkle in his eye. After that I thought no more of the incident.

But once I returned home he kept pestering me: 'I want to come to Park Hospital. I want to see what you're doing. I want to learn from you.' On it went. So along he came, accompanied by his glamorous wife Rina. I thought this would shut him up but it only increased his persistence. 'I want you to set up IVF clinic in Rome and a chain around Italy – you can do whatever you like there and be a superstar!'

I wasn't interested in superstardom but I was definitely attracted by the research and development opportunities Antinori was dangling in front of me. Looking into his background, I discovered he was an obstetrician and gynaecologist who hadn't worked with IVF but who obviously wanted to learn more about it. Crucially he was also prepared to let me develop SUZI at his clinic in Rome, which meant I could prove it was safe one way or the other without the restrictions placed on me in the UK. I asked Malcolm Symonds if he'd heard of this chap. He hadn't but kindly contacted some of his international colleagues on my behalf to make sure I wasn't leaping out of the frying pan into the fire. The feedback was that Antinori was a somewhat strange and crazy guy, but that as long as I kept control of my notes and my work there was no reason why I shouldn't grab this opportunity. The hospital and university gave their blessing for me to combine my work there with the clinical and research work in Italy. This meant I'd added a third job to my workload – it was going to be a busy few years.

I agreed with Antinori we'd take things slowly at first, with me travelling to Rome for a mixture of short weekends in which I'd undertake four or five cases, and long weekends in which I'd handle ten or fifteen. Our first clinic was part of a private hospital north of the city known as 'Villa Claudia', in which he'd built a spanking new IVF unit with all the equipment I desired. If I asked for the finest micro-manipulators by a particular company, or the most modern incubators available, it was 'nessun problema' (no problem). What a contrast to the university, where even getting a cup and saucer meant filling in a requisition form. Ever ambitious, he soon set about expanding into a group of clinics and asked me to bring in international colleagues from Sweden, Canada, the US, Australia, and Germany to act as figureheads and provide a governing body to approve new research. I became 'Presidente' of the group, which we called RAPRU (Ricercatori Associati Perla Riproduzione Umana [Association for Research into Human Reproduction]). Remember there was at that time no official IVF regulation anywhere in the world, let alone in Italy, which had a reputation as being a bit of the Wild West of IVF at that time (although today it's swung the other way and has become ridiculously over-regulated).

I finally had the opportunity to prove SUZI was safe. And it was tough because I had three jobs: one managing a huge case load in Italy, one at the university back home, and one at the Park Clinic in Nottingham. The SUZI work in Rome, which I had to undertake with no assistance, meant sixteen- to twenty-hour days to complete the patient load. Sometimes I'd be away from home for three weeks at a time, with forty-eight hours back home before I turned myself around again. I'd regularly collect multiple eggs from as many as seven patients in one day, ending up with a huge number to fertilise by injection which had to be done before I left Rome at the end of the weekend. There was no protocol for the procedure – I was establishing it from scratch.

My frantic schedule meant I barely saw my family, and things came to a head in 1988 when my father became seriously ill. Knowing he might be dying, but also aware I had my busiest ever run of patients coming up in Rome, I asked his specialist if it was sensible for me to travel. How long was he likely to live, I wanted to know. 'At least six months, Simon', he told me. 'Don't worry – off you go.' So I went, and planned to spend the next ten days with the ninety patients on my list. After two days I received a call from my brother-in-law telling me Dad had died and immediately flew home. At that time I was trialling a brand-new drug which controlled women's menstrual cycles, which meant we could stop ovulation while I was at home and start it again when I was able to travel to the clinic on my weekends. There was nothing for it but to apply the drug now, with Antinori keeping most of the ninety patients on hold until I'd gone to the funeral and back.

It was all worth it, though, because in 1990 I finally achieved the world's first birth using SUZI: a baby girl, Maria Russo. The night of her birth was one of the most nerve-wracking of my life because we'd agreed ITN could film it alongside a live broadcast by Italian TV station Rai Uno, which was like the BBC over there. The experience gave me a glimpse into how Bob and Patrick must have felt when the birth of Louise Brown was broadcast. Part of the reason it was so worrying was because specialists carried out a detailed ultrasound scan, and shortly before the big day Antinori had phoned me with the terrible news the baby had Hirschsprung's disease, a congenital condition which affects the large intestine. This was all we needed. I couldn't see how the problem had anything to do with SUZI but I seriously considered cancelling the filming. In the end we held our nerve and I flew to Italy in the morning to attend the delivery that night with cameras present. During the day I remember standing on the Ponte Vecchio in Rome beside myself with despair, because this birth was going to be shown to the world and I'd wanted so much to prove it was safe.

Maria Russo was born with ITN and Rai Uno filming every step of the way, and the ultrasound turned out to be wrong. Thank God! She was normal, healthy, and fine, and I have a lovely photo of me holding her which I treasure to this day. I was delighted to have shown SUZI was without problems, and in order to get the data out into the scientific community I published my research in *The Lancet* later that year.[9]

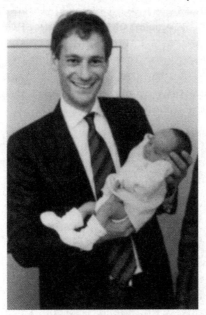

Figure 4.4: Maria Russo

As well as being hugely satisfying on a personal level, this case was a critical turning point in my career because I became known for achieving a significant breakthrough in fertility treatment, especially for male-factor conditions. It was certainly instrumental in me being offered the opportunity for my next venture. Having said that, although SUZI was safe it wasn't terribly successful. In Italy we only achieved a five to 10 per cent live birth rate with it, depending on the age of the patient. There were still many couples who wanted to give it a go, though, because without it they were either going to have a success rate of zero or would have to use donor sperm.

While I was in Italy I took the opportunity of giving a live demonstration of SUZI on Rai Uno, the Italian television channel, and while I was doing so displayed a related technique I'd developed in my spare moments there. This was to inject the sperm directly into the egg, rather than just the space between the outer shell and the egg. I explained I would only ever do

---

[9]   Fishel, Antinori et al. 1990.

this on a test egg for research because it was hugely invasive and I wasn't sure of the effect on the resulting embryo, but I already had a name for it. It was DISCO (Direct Injection of the Sperm into the Cytoplasm of the Oocyte). Little was I to know that four or five years later this method would be achieved accidentally (a story for another time), but my demonstration on Rai Uno did net me the Fregene Award, an annual Italian prize for the person who makes an impact at an international level through the use of communication.

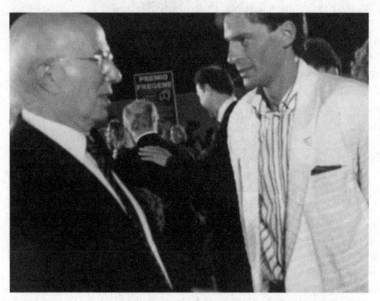

Figure 4.5: Meeting Renato Dulbecco, 1975 Nobel Prize in Physiology or Medicine winner at the Fregene Awards

When I and my team developed SUZI we took a blind leap of faith, and like everything I've introduced into IVF over the years it attracted an element of antagonism, with comments such as 'it's a slippery slope' and 'what will these mad Frankenstein doctors do next?' Today 60 to 70 per cent of IVF cases are treated by sperm micro-injection, although they don't all require it – it's simply more efficient that way. Many US clinics use it for *all* their patients.

During the three years Antinori and I worked together I gained a fascinating – and at times terrifying – insight into his character. The risk-taking approach that had attracted me in the first place, along with his drive and energy, started to backfire when his clinics became successful and his fame spread. He had an unbelievably large PR machine following him around to promote his work, which led to him becoming enormously well known and phenomenally wealthy. Eventually he started to believe he was some kind of untouchable genius and became increasingly violent and aggressive. One time, when I was beginning to question the integrity of his work, we had a huge row and he grabbed a heavy wrench and started smashing the container in which the patients' frozen embryos were stored. I also witnessed him hurl an uncapped syringe at an anaesthetist across a patient on the operating table. It got to the point at which I had to tell him I couldn't work with him anymore. It was obvious to me he was furious, but he made an attempt to control himself, saying 'Attenzione. Aspetta. (You wait)', before marching out of the room. Hanging around was the last thing I intended to do, and I immediately started packing up my belongings in the clinic. At this point a heavy hand landed on my shoulder from behind. Turning around, I saw his extremely large nephew who often ran errands for him in front of me.

'Siediti (Sit down)', he ordered. 'You wait here until Severino returns.'

As I started to explain in Italian what I was doing, I could see arguing was pointless and given he was twice my size I judged it prudent to do as I was told. I waited a full two hours until Antinori returned waving a piece of paper: 'Simon, sign this.' The document was a hastily drawn-up contract stating I wouldn't work for anyone else in IVF ever again. Naturally I protested, but he grew increasingly agitated: 'Sign it! Sign it!'

The next thing he did I have trouble believing even now: he took out a gun and put it to my temple. 'Otherwise, I kill you.'

Needless to say I signed the contract, packed my bags, and made a swift exit as he cried out after me, 'A domani (see you tomorrow)!' Running to a phone box in the street, I called Judy. 'Do me a favour and don't ask any questions. Just get our luggage and I'll see you at the airport. We're leaving.'

After I left Antinori I was nervous about returning to Italy, because although his bark was worse than his bite, it was still pretty terrible! I even wondered if he'd turn up at my front door at home one day. Never was the psychotic element of his personality more evident than during a BBC-filmed debate with Robert Winston which took place some time after my departure. Antinori had started to treat women in their 60s with egg donation (the practice which eventually made him infamous), and Winston had been invited to discuss the ethics of it with him. It ended up being the most amazing piece of television I've ever seen. Winston was a huge critic of Antinori's, and one thing I'll say about Antinori was that he always took critics head on. The interview started with the interviewer sitting on his own in my old office at the Rome clinic, introducing the two opponents before they strode in as if they were gladiators. No sooner had they sat down than Antinori jumped up, went across to Winston, and jabbed his finger in his face.

'Are you Arab? You're Arab, aren't you?' he said. 'Get out of my clinic!'

The result was a fracas, culminating in Antinori grabbing the BBC camera and throwing it down a flight of stairs. The scene then cut to Winston outside on the street in front of the clinic, visibly shaking. 'I came to discuss with Antinori whether he should be treating older women. I've come to the conclusion he shouldn't be allowed to treat anyone at all', he said. Hilariously the TV programme made the front page of the Italian newspapers with the headline, 'Hoodlum sent by Thatcher from Britain to destroy Antinori's clinic'. It turned out Antinori had semi-wrecked his own office by throwing chairs and papers everywhere and had then brought in the media to show 'what Winston has done to my clinic'.

Despite my Italian adventure taking up a fair amount of my time and energy, I still spent most of this time carrying out my research and clinical responsibilities in Nottingham. In 1986 I worked on a fascinating case, that of Susan Ooi, who I'm still in touch with today. She was a Chinese woman living in England who came to the Park Clinic for IVF. Because of her condition I couldn't collect any eggs from her so the only way she could have a baby was to use someone else's. We had our own Park Hospital ethics committee by this time, which was completely independent, and one of the first IVF ethics committees ever established; I had captivating debates with them on many occasions. As in every case like this, I assessed the couple and asked the committee's view. My opinion, and that of my colleagues, was that in this particular instance egg donation could only be beneficial if from family members, who were fully aware of what they were embarking on. The committee agreed we could bring Susan's sister over from New York for an egg donation, synchronising the two women to undertake a fresh embryo transfer but also freezing any remaining embryos. After the embryo transfer in November 1986, Susan became pregnant but had an early miscarriage. When she returned we built up the lining of her womb with oestrogen and progesterone and transferred two frozen embryos on Saturday 7 March 1987. This time it worked and she became pregnant with twins, which were delivered on 21 September after 28 weeks' gestation. Susan and her husband John called the boys Robin (after Robin Hood – the clinic was near Sherwood Forest) and Simon (very kindly, after me).

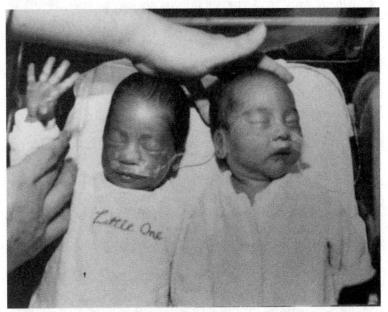

Figure 4.6: The Ooi twins as babies

Because of this case being that of the world's first twins born from frozen embryos created by donated eggs, it generated a lot of publicity; and because we also had to undertake an unusual sperm preparation and insemination procedure it was dubbed the most 'hi-tech' pregnancy of our time. As I'd come to expect by then, I was pilloried by scientific circles for carrying out an egg donation by a donor known to its recipient. 'Who are you to determine who these children's mother is?' was an example line. 'And if they're allowed to identify the donor – in this case their aunt – how do you know what pain could be unleashed?' As it happens, I recently met my namesake Simon for the first time. It was wonderful to see him and he invited me to his forthcoming wedding – how lovely. For me it felt of historic importance to have a frank conversation with him after all these years, about how he felt growing up in unusual circumstances. He was clear his aunt was his aunt, not his mother, and the family was close and happy. Clearly they've all done a wonderful job.

The HFEA wasn't yet established so it was decided by the acting regulators that in future only anonymous donations should be allowed (although they didn't ban sister-to-sister egg donation). This was until 2005, when it was eventually decided by the HFEA that *all* donors should be identifiable to the conceived child after the age of eighteen, although not to the recipient at the time of donation. Such is the strange world of regulation. Now sister-to-sister egg donation is relatively commonplace, and even daughter-to-mother or vice versa. As for Robin and Simon, they live happy lives and Susan regularly sends me pictures of them, always expressing her gratitude. So it was a brilliant outcome, despite the enormous concerns about the 'terrible' thing I'd done to this family!

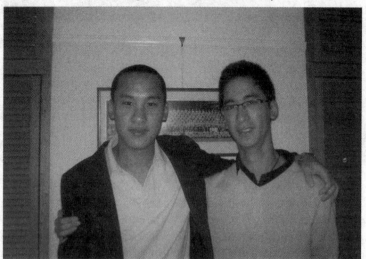

Figure 4.7: The Ooi twins as young men

This wasn't the only controversial treatment we pioneered. I received a visit from a woman whose daughters had galactosaemia, a disease that used to be life-threatening but that by now could be managed fairly successfully through diet. However, because for some reason the ovaries are exquisitely sensitive to galactosaemia, women with it progress to menopause shortly after puberty which limits their fertility. This mother wanted me to freeze her own eggs so she could donate them to her girls when they were older. I told her I'd love to help but that I didn't have the right technology. However, I wrote to a galactosaemia expert in the US called Professor Kauffman to ask if a woman with this condition could carry a pregnancy with a donated egg. She said she thought it would be possible, which meant we'd be able to freeze eggs and use them for women like these daughters. At least that way their babies would come from within their own family line. In the end it did turn out to be a condition that was amenable to egg donation, and eighteen years later we carried out the first donor egg IVF to a woman with galactosaemia. This is one of the joys of living through such changes in technology.

When I think about it, my whole career has involved coming up against a series of brick walls and working out ways to get over them. I've constantly asked myself, 'what technology do I need to develop or is there one already in another field that I can latch onto?' One of the things I've learned is that once a new development is proven to work, more and different types of patients hear about it and ask for it. That's why IVF has so much impact today. If we could only offer people what we originally could at the start of the Bourn Hall days, it would be a seriously niche activity restricted to married women with fallopian tube problems.

Times were moving on. In 1990, parliament voted to allow IVF to continue as a practice by passing the Human Fertilisation and Embryology Act; this gave rise to the Human Fertilisation and Embryology Authority (HFEA), the regulatory body for the IVF industry. Its first chairman happened to be Professor Sir Colin Campbell, the Vice Chancellor of Nottingham University, and therefore my university employer.

Some time after the passing of the Act, Malcolm Symonds came to me saying that he had spoken with Campbell, who had told him that if I still wanted an academic IVF facility in the university, I now could because parliament had ratified IVF. He said that as he was the first chair of the HFEA, he himself would have to take a back seat, but when the Bursar and other senior academics had set up the appropriate arrangements and contracts, then I could go ahead.

I was at a crossroads. In many ways this was a dream come true because I was being offered on a plate what I'd striven for since I was at Cambridge: a fully integrated research and clinical department – a beacon of an academic institution with international standing that would drive IVF forward. On the other hand, the Park Hospital clinic had thousands of patients and a fantastic team including John and Peter; I didn't relish leaving everything I'd built up there. After agonising over it for a long time though, I had to admit that carrying on at the Park clinic wasn't my dream. My vision was to set up a teaching course to train IVF practitioners, with the obvious benefit of having all the material to carry out a combined IVF clinic and research facility under one roof. I also wanted to be associated with an NHS fertility clinic, both physically and politically, so I could do more for NHS patients. It was hard to have one part of our work at the Park Hospital's private facility and another at the university; when I needed to shift gametes and embryos, for instance, I had to move them across town. And if I'd wanted to set up a degree course, or even a short-term training course, the students couldn't come to the Park Hospital to gain practical experience because the facilities weren't there. I'd even written to Richard Branson with the tongue-in-cheek suggestion that he fund the set-up of a 'Virgin Institute of Fertility', but to no avail.

I took a deep breath and announced to John that I was moving away from the Park Clinic to set up in opposition at the university. He was obviously upset but his only words to me were that if I really wanted it, then I must do it. Inevitably we would become competitors in a small marketplace, although it was an ever expanding one as global demand for IVF was increasing all the time. As I sat in my office at the hospital with Malcolm one Saturday morning while he was prepping for his private operations that day, a name for the new clinic came to me. He loved it too. I was to call it NURTURE: Nottingham University Research and Treatment Unit in Reproduction. The ground-breaking Nurture years were about to begin, although they were to end in a way I could thankfully never have foreseen.

Chapter 5
The Nurture Years
1991–1997

My years at Nurture were some of the most fulfilling of my career. Together with my team I was able to pretty much double the number of people I could help by developing more techniques to help infertile men as well as women. I helped spread high-level IVF expertise around the world through my degree programme, and I created a profitable and successful clinic. This period was, however, also filled with the most frustrating and traumatic events I've ever experienced.

In some ways, things started off much the same as when I'd commuted to Italy for Antinori, in that I spent the next twelve months shuttling back and forth to Rome. Being under a restricted covenant from the Park Hospital meant I wasn't allowed to work at Nurture for a year, although I could still carry on my teaching and research at Nottingham University. Concerned I might lose my sperm micro-injection skills in the meanwhile, I was glad to be asked by some Italian colleagues from my Antinori days, Doctors Lisi and Rinaldi, if I could help them set up their own IVF clinic there.

During that time in Italy I gave a talk on the island of Elba about sperm micro-injection. It was to an international audience so I was determined to make a good impression. Disaster struck when I arrived at my hotel on the Friday afternoon ready for my talk on the Saturday, only to unpack my case and find to my horror I'd left my slides at home. There was no way I could cobble together a new set on the spot, nor could I face such an eminent audience without visual aids. In full panic mode I managed to locate a shop and buy some overhead acetates and pens. Rushing back to my room, I grabbed the phone and dialled my office number, offering up a silent thank you as my call was answered by a somewhat disgruntled secretary who was still in the office. I directed her to my desk and asked her to describe every single slide in painstaking detail while I sketched them out on the acetates; I'll be forever grateful for her patience. When I gave the talk it was so embarrassing. I had no real proof I'd done anything at all, because I had no photographs of my tools or the eggs under the microscope – all I had were my terrible drawings and the data I'd conjured up from memory.

My Italian work kept me busy until I was eventually able to open Nurture in August 1991. A pivotal point earlier that year had been the formation of the HFEA, the regulatory body for the IVF industry, and its first meeting to which I'd been invited along with practitioners from other IVF clinics. Most of the conference was pretty dull but a single sentence from one of the new regulators made me prick up my ears: 'It's going to take us at least a year to inspect all IVF clinics and establish our Code of Practice; until that time you can continue as you are.' In other words, until the HFEA inspected us Nurture would be free of regulation! I almost had to stop myself from rubbing my hands with glee. My expertise in SUZI was the golden egg that would safeguard Nurture's future, but so far I'd not been allowed to practice it in the UK. Now I had a precious window of opportunity in which to prove it effective and safe on home soil – an opportunity that would, after a year, slam shut. Given Nurture hadn't yet opened its doors, I did some hasty mental arithmetic and rushed back to put a proposal in front of Malcolm.

'We have to double the speed of the unit's launch and get it up and running in three months', I said. 'The HFEA regulators are bound to make us one of the first they inspect. If we launch early we can beat them to it. If not, we're done for. We have to get practising SUZI before they visit us.'

So that's what we did, because although I wasn't allowed to work at Nurture until my restricted covenant was spent I could still get the ball rolling. I spent months harassing the estates management department at the university to open the facility, and my wife Judy and I got it up and running between us – we even slept there some nights. This resulted in us opening ahead of schedule and I started my first SUZI cases straight away.

Our first SUZI success, in 1992, was for a lovely couple whose baby was in effect Britain's Maria Russo. The family was featured on the front page of the *Daily Mail* ('Meet James the First') and the story went international, pinning Nurture on the map from the beginning and allowing us to steal a march on other IVF clinics. If I hadn't attended that HFEA meeting, the start of Nurture might have been radically different.

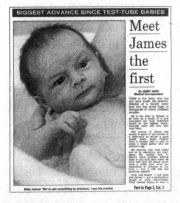

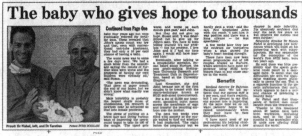

Figure 5.1: 'Meet James the First', *Daily Mail*, 7 September 1992

After this I was constantly looking for ways to improve SUZI by making the penetration of the egg's outer shell easier. My challenge was to ensure this process was smooth, but without creating any pressure points that would damage the fragile egg by hitting the membrane. One day I came across a technology using what's known as the 'piezoelectric effect', which means applying a vibration to the needle that's so finely tuned it's barely perceptible but still allowing a stabbing motion so the needle passes through the shell. The aim was to make it similar to a knife cutting through butter. I called this the 'Sonic Sword' and published an article about it in 1994.[10]

James's case was the first of several world-first successes at Nurture. The next was the first 'sugar-drop' frozen embryo baby later that year, a development that was borne of my desire to make the embryo freezing process more reliable and a lot cheaper. The traditional way of freezing an embryo was to embalm it in a kind of biological antifreeze before putting it into a freezer. This entailed an expensive, computerised machine pumping liquid nitrogen into a reservoir at a precise rate of a third of a degree per minute. The painstakingly slow reduction in temperature took three or four hours to complete, and no matter how carefully it was carried out it contained the risk of ice crystals damaging the cytoplasm inside the cells. To make this quicker and more reliable we developed a new solution to replace the antifreeze. This rapidly removed the water from the cell and made it almost glass-like, after which we could plunge the embryo straight into the liquid nitrogen without delay. The glassy appearance gave rise to the scientific name of 'vitrification', although 'sugar-drop' was what it was popularly called. The new technique reduced the cost of freezing by tens of thousands of pounds, because it didn't require such expensive technology and reduced the time from hours to minutes. Once we were sure it was safe we applied to the HFEA for permission to carry it out clinically, describing the full process. To our delight we were given permission to go ahead.

Our first successful case of freezing an embryo using this technique was that of Maureen Hogarth, who was over the moon when she discovered she was pregnant. In October 1992 she gave birth to her daughter Laura. Maureen and her husband Andrew attracted quite a bit of media attention because of the innovative nature of this embryo freezing, which didn't escape the HFEA. As I was in my office reading a scientific journal my phone rang. It was one of the HFEA staff members, asking me what on earth I thought I was up to. Apparently, I was in serious

---

[10]   Proceedings of the European Workshop on Micromanipulation of Gametes and Embryos and Symposium', Brussels, December 1993, 'Advantages of the Use of the Sonic Sword in Micromanipulation of Gametes and Embryos'; Fishel, Timson et al. 1993.

trouble for carrying out a process that hadn't been sanctioned by them.

'But you gave it the go-ahead', I replied, frantically digging out the paperwork from my desk drawer. 'You wrote and told me I could do it. I have it here in front of me.' There was a long silence on the other end of the line, which was eventually broken by a promise to come back to me. I had a nervous wait, but eventually the HFEA wrote to tell me that because I'd informed it about the sugar-drop process I wouldn't be censured. However, it was still placing a moratorium on it. The explanation? 'We didn't realise it was so new.'

So that was vitrification finished. A technique that would have made freezing embryos, and therefore IVF, both cheaper, quicker, and more reliable, was condemned to the archives because it was 'too new' for the HFEA back in 1992. About ten years ago, however, it slowly crept back into use because other scientists could see it made sense; it's now mainstream, despite the HFEA never having officially lifted its ban. This is the way the HFEA often works. Its objectives shuffle around every time a new Chair is appointed, accompanied by new aims and mantras. As for Laura, she's now graduated from university and is a normal, healthy woman. It's a shame about the HFEA ban because there were many more who could have come after her if the regulators hadn't made freezing embryos hugely more expensive than it needed to be.

In 1994 we developed another ground-breaking technology, which resulted in the world's first baby born due to CISS (Computer Image Sperm Selection). Essentially it was a way of making SUZI more effective and involved us working with – of all people – an engineering professor called Geoff Hobson, who'd created a new way of monitoring traffic movements on the motorway. We knew sperm had three characteristics: the way the head twitches from side to side, the path the sperm takes, and the thrashing of the tail (or 'hyperactivated motion'). The 'thrashers' were the best at fertilising an egg, and with SUZI being such a painstaking process it made sense to select only the most hyperactivated sperm to inject so we could maximise the number of eggs we could fertilise. The problem was how to find them. There was no way of detecting the thrashers simply by looking at them under a microscope, so we had to find a way of recognising the most useful sperm so we could pick them out.

I asked my colleague Steve Green to approach Geoff, to see if his computerised image scanner could count and analyse the precise movement of individual sperm as well as it did with traffic, and also give us a way of visually selecting them. Geoff said he didn't see why not and that he'd give it a go. We worked on this technology together and he was able to develop a colour coding system to denote sperm by their quality of movement that was invisible to the human eye. This meant while the sperm were under the microscope we could simultaneously observe on a monitor those that were in a state of readiness to fertilise an egg, by viewing a white tracking line. By watching the monitor and making tiny precision movements with our micro-manipulator we could guide the needle to pick up the best sperm, each measuring only five millionths of a metre. This, along with our Sonic Sword, helped us increase our fertilisation rates considerably. What was so exciting about this development was the fusion between IVF and other disciplines, engineers having been instrumental in the development of both SUZI and CISS. I said to Steve, 'This will be your PhD.' And it was.

Although CISS was cutting edge, it was quickly overtaken by a new development, this time instigated by an Italian friend of mine living in Brussels, Gianpiero Palermo. We bumped into each other at a conference in New York some years later, and while we were standing in a doorway getting some air he confided in me. 'Do you know, I'm ever so grateful to you Simon because I'd never have had success with ICSI if you hadn't developed SUZI first.' I'd heard about his ICSI work and was keen to know the details as they'd never been made clear, so pressed him for more information. He explained he'd been carrying out a fertilisation using SUZI when the needle accidentally slipped and he mistakenly injected the sperm into the centre of the egg, rather than the safer zona pellucida just inside the shell. Withdrawing the needle, he'd assumed the egg's cytoplasm would leak out and it would die, but it didn't – the sperm stayed in and the shell remained intact. Surprised, he tried it a few more times and achieved an excellent fertilisation rate; in fact, of the eggs that survived the process, 70 per cent became fertilised. Compare that to SUZI's success rate, which was at that time running at 25 per cent. Palermo decided to call it Intracytoplasmic Sperm Injection, or ICSI. I admired his courage because even I hadn't dared to carry out a procedure more invasive than SUZI, and yet he had made it work (how he managed to acquire ethical approval to carry it out in Belgium at the time, is another story).

I was puzzled, though. Given I knew scientists around the world had been unsuccessfully trying for years to achieve exactly what Palermo had succeeded in doing, what explained his positive results? This question led me to return yet again to Rome, because carrying out this kind of research was still not something I could do at home. I instigated a huge project in which I took sibling eggs (it was essential they were from the same woman) and kept them in the same environment but tried fertilising them using different methods of ICSI. My experimentation taught me there were two critical elements to making the process highly successful. One was to cut the tail of the sperm to stop it moving before injecting it into the egg, so as to replicate what happens naturally (once a sperm fuses with the membrane of the egg it's grasped and pulled in, immobilising the tail). This was tricky because I had to locate the tail and cut it when it was microscopically small. The second was, before injecting the sperm, to 'invaginate' the inner egg membrane by sucking it up into a tiny pipette twelve times thinner than a human hair. The skill lay in allowing the pipette's sharp point to then gently tear through the egg membrane, but without causing the cytoplasm inside to spill out and destroy it. Once the pipette was withdrawn, the membrane rapidly re-sealed.

Why was this important? Because the membrane of an egg is elastic, like the surface of a balloon. Many practitioners were pushing the needle into it thinking they were then getting inside the egg, but in fact they were only causing an invagination. When they injected the sperm and retracted the pipette, the membrane would re-form and eject the sperm straight back into the culture medium. This obviously meant the egg remained unfertilised because the sperm had never penetrated it. Eventually I developed a machine that could kill the pressure in the pipette as soon as I saw a rush of cytoplasm about to start, which minimised damage to the egg. These two discoveries meant I was able to achieve an extraordinarily high success rate almost overnight.

To share what I'd learned I submitted a paper to the respected journal *Human Reproduction*, set up and run by Bob Edwards. Publication was delayed for an awfully long time, and when I eventually saw my article in print I laughed with incredulity.[11] On one page was my article, and on the next was a piece by Antinori which described that same experiment. Scientific ideas and processes can of course be conceived around the same time, but I could see the names associated with the Antinori paper were not those of people who could ever have performed those techniques. It will forever remain a mystery as reviewing scientific manuscripts is, and always has been, an anonymous process – almost shrouded in secrecy – so I couldn't gain any further information. As many years have gone by now, I thought I might finally be able to find out what happened: was there skulduggery or was I being paranoid? I asked the editor to dig back into the dusty archives for me but they only go back as far as when digital copies were stored. So I'll never get to the bottom of it, which is a pity as we scientists place a lot of store by historical accuracy.

These innovations in sperm injection were transformative. SUZI, CISS, and eventually ICSI (which rendered both the former unnecessary), allowed 95 per cent of men with sperm problems presenting for treatment to become genetic fathers, even if those problems were extreme. Never again were they made to choose between childlessness and using donor sperm – it was a revolution.

Because at Nurture we were the first in the UK to offer sperm injection technology, by the mid-1990s we were receiving an enormous number of requests from other clinics asking us to teach them how to do it. I knew I couldn't help them all myself so I said to Malcolm, who was my Head of Department, 'What if we were to ask some of our star embryology performers to help?' Ken Dowell was an obstetrician and gynaecologist working with us and he could teach others the medical aspects (he's still my colleague today). Malcolm thought this was a great idea.

'Do it', he said. 'It's great for the university, it's great for Nurture, and it will get ICSI more widely known. You have carte blanche to go ahead.' So I and my team travelled to Cairo, Rome, the Middle East, and many other cities and countries to train practitioners not only in IVF but also in our emerging technologies such as sperm micro-injection. The advantage to

---

[11]   Fishel, Lisi et al. 1995.

us was that, given the restrictions on research and development in the UK, we had the opportunity to try out our ideas abroad instead. After all, it was working in Rome with SUZI that had kept us ahead of the game in the early days of regulation.

Nurture wasn't all about the research and practice of IVF, though. One of my ambitions when I'd first started was to set up a post-graduate IVF degree course and after a hectic first year establishing the clinic, I managed to launch it. We called it a Master's degree in ART (Assisted Reproduction Technology) or, as one local TV station coined it, the world's first degree course in making babies. Working with Dr Steven Fleming, who I'd appointed as a lecturer for the purpose, we created not only a template for other universities to use later, but a wealth of research through our graduate theses. We received applications from over ninety countries in the first few months, resulting in my first group of British and international students, some of whom became lifelong friends. It was their first opportunity to gain in-depth knowledge and hands-on experience, and to take back high-tech IVF to their own countries. Every day was a brave new world to them; they'd only ever heard about this kind of technology before, and some of them were lucky enough to be there when we treated patients who were world-first cases for us too. Because of the way it ran I spent most of my Christmases marking exam papers and dissertations. Despite that, I revelled in it as a wonderfully academic and generative period of my life, in many ways re-capturing the excitement of my early years at Bourn Hall. It also gave us the opportunity to learn together and expand our field, and it was lucrative for the university because most of the students were foreign and so paid double the fees of those from the UK.

As well as welcoming students from abroad I did a lot of travelling myself. One of my most memorable trips was to the island of Ischia in Italy. I'd been invited to open a conference there, accompanied by my wife Judy and our baby son Bobby. The plan was for me to give the keynote speech on the first evening, after which a gala dinner would be served. Unfortunately, we only got as far as the local airport when things started to go wrong as we missed our flight due to a hold-up at security. I could even see the plane through the boarding gate window: 'Is that our plane?' I begged, 'Please let me on. We *have* to get this flight.' But no. Eventually we made it to Naples via at least two other airports, where we were met by a taxi arranged by the conference organisers who were desperate for me to make it in time. Needless to say, the traffic in Naples was appalling and we arrived at the ferry port only to see our boat to Ischia chugging merrily off into the distance. The driver informed us that if we didn't want to wait four hours for the next one, we had to dash to another port from which an alternative ferry would be departing in ten minutes. I covered my eyes as he reversed us down a four-lane highway at top speed with my wife and baby in the back, and we arrived at the venue exhausted and drenched in sweat. There was no smiling welcome committee, though. Here was a fabulous gala dinner about to be served on the beautiful outside terraces of the hotel, and I'd kept everyone waiting for two hours. The chefs alone were livid. 'I'll just change into my suit', I said.

'No. Now. *Subito*', was the reply. So I went ahead with my talk in my jeans and t-shirt (although at least I had my slides, unlike in Elba).

It was a time of tumultuous change throughout Europe, as well as within the scientific world. As Eastern Europe liberated itself from the shackles of Communism, we started to receive more visitors from Russia. One day out of the blue, a lady by the name of Mrs Popova arrived in my office with her grown-up daughter. Mrs Popova couldn't speak much English but she was able to say 'My daughter needs your help.' The daughter had no way of paying for treatment, but, ever keen to help those who wouldn't normally be able to afford it, I persuaded a drug company to supply the medication free of charge, and we carried out IVF for her. Several months later I was delighted to receive a letter from the Soviet Union thanking me for my help. Mrs Popover's daughter had given birth to twins, naming them Mikhail and Elizabeth after the 'glorious leaders' of our countries: Mikhail Gorbachev and Her Majesty Queen Elizabeth. She described how humanity had moved on with the new openness in the East, and how lucky she'd been to be able to travel to our country, a pioneer of IVF technology. I was tickled by this and forwarded a copy of the letter to Buckingham Palace together with a photograph of the twins. Apparently, her Majesty was 'most pleased' with it and I have her reply on my office wall today.

In 1996 I received a visit from a lovely couple called Gavin and Jenny 'O'. Their fertility problem, and our solution to it, turned out to be one of the most fascinating I've ever come across. It was also to turn one of my colleagues' hair grey. At this time it was often hard for patients to find their way to us because most doctors and specialists, even in the fertility field, didn't know we could help solve male infertility problems as well as female ones. That's why some, like the Os, found us through the media. They'd been trying for a baby for years but had been told it would never work because Gavin wasn't able to produce sperm. As it happened we were beginning to re-write the text books on this topic because we were discovering so many new things, such as the long-held belief that sperm in the testes were not necessarily immotile as had previously been assumed. I explained to Gavin and Jenny that occasionally I could find sperm by a method I had developed while working in Italy with men who had similar conditions; I called it Multiple Ejaculations Resuspension and Centrifugation, or MERC. This involved asking the man to ejaculate two or three times in one day if possible, and then washing and concentrating the seminal plasma down into a fraction of a teardrop. Once the sperm had then been separated out using a sedimentation solution, I'd sometimes be able to find a single sperm or two in a man who'd been told he didn't have any. Gavin agreed we could do this procedure and we arranged to carry it out once we'd primed his wife Jenny to produce eggs.

When a man starts to manufacture sperm it takes about seventy days to grow from a stem cell to what I like to think of as a fully formed, magical thing called sperm. A grown-up sperm is only a single cell, but it's undergone the most amazing transformation by the time it's mature. It gains two parts to its head: the area containing the DNA it will pass to the egg and a 'cap', which is a sac containing enzymes that digest a hole in the egg's outer shell to help the sperm drive through into the perivitelline space. It also has a neck that contains the centriole; this is important for the tail movement and also to help the chromosomes to divide when they eventually enter the egg. In addition this neck contains the batteries, or mitochondria, that provide the power to propel the tail through its different motions. Finally there's the tail, which is fifty millionths of a metre long. In conventional reproduction, not only has this tail to push the sperm head through the outer shell, but also to propel the sperm to the site of the egg membrane so the sperm can fertilise the egg.

When the time came for us to examine Gavin's sperm one Friday morning, I was disappointed – after a couple of hours preparing the samples and searching them – to find only a few spermatids. These are immature male sex cells that may develop into a sperm – in other words, they're still a couple of stages before the end of the sperm maturation process. His had short tails and were not fully developed, although I thought the heads seemed normal so there should be no problem with their DNA. I felt it was important the couple knew the full reality of the situation so I said to them, 'Unfortunately this is all I've got. I've no idea if it can fertilise your eggs because it's never been done before – I just don't know. The options are: we don't do it because we don't know what the outcome will be, or we do it, see if fertilisation occurs, and then have another chat.' I also told them I'd have to inform the HFEA, but that as it was now the weekend I wouldn't be able to contact them until Monday.

Their response was clear. 'We know it's cutting-edge technology', they said, 'and there are risks involved. But please go ahead and try to fertilise the eggs. If you're happy with what the embryo looks like we'd like it transferred.'

Returning to the lab on Saturday, I was astonished to see one egg was fertilised. I told the couple, who were thrilled, but warned them it would probably not divide. To my amazement, by Sunday it had divided into two cells and was approaching the stage when it would be ready to be transferred. Before I could do so I needed clarity from the HFEA, so I said to Gavin and Jenny, 'If the worst comes to the worst and the HFEA can't give its view tomorrow, we'll freeze your embryo until the regulator tells me what I'm allowed to do.' In those days frozen wasn't as good as fresh, so I much preferred to work with a fresh embryo.

First thing on Monday morning I called the regulator to request an urgent decision. The man I spoke to wasn't happy. I was told that I had put the HFEA on the spot by announcing a new development before they'd had time to discuss it. They told me to do what I thought best for my patient and that afterwards they would consider it more fully. The line was that that for now I must make my own judgement and seek my own legal advice. Unfortunately that's always the way the HFEA works; it likes to avoid taking responsibility for as many decisions as possible.

'So I can do what I think is best for the patient?' I confirmed. They agreed I could.

I'd recently appointed a medical director to Nurture, Simon Thornton (he eventually became my business partner and friend, although he's recently retired – considerably younger than me – to become a game ranger in Africa). After he joined me he confessed he'd received a good-natured warning about me beforehand: 'If you're going to take this medical directorship at Nurture, just be aware Fishel's on the edge. He likes to work at the limits of what's possible.' I took that as a compliment and we became friends straightaway. After talking him through the Os' case I agreed with him we'd go ahead with the embryo transfer because the HFEA had given us carte blanche to do what was best for the patient. We carried out the transfer and, as always, said a quiet prayer that it would succeed although we weren't optimistic in this case.

Just over two weeks later Simon called me with the news Jenny was pregnant. You can imagine our surprise and delight. However, as we knew only too well, a chemical test of pregnancy is a long way from confirming a baby was growing in the womb. I didn't want to let myself get too excited; indeed, there was much at stake because not only would there be the normal hurdles facing any pregnant mother at such an early stage, but the outcome of this conception was unknown to medical science. My fears were partially allayed when at six weeks an ultrasound scan confirmed the pregnancy and we could see it was developing well. I wrote a hasty scientific paper, had it reviewed by its co-authors, and submitted it to The Lancet. This was (and still is) a prestigious journal, and the very same one in which Bob and Patrick had published their seminal 'Birth after the reimplantation of a human embryo' on 12 October 1978.[12] At the same time I updated the HFEA and headed off to Ibiza for a much-needed holiday.

There was soon to be trouble in paradise. While I was on my sun lounger I received a call from Simon Thornton to tell me there was trouble afoot with the HFEA. I immediately called them and received a chilling response: Nurture was now in deep trouble and was in danger of losing its licence to practice. An internal meeting was being convened to discuss whether we would be forced to close, but if I was to take the decision

---

[12] Steptoe PC, Edwards, RG. Birth after reimplantation of a human embryo, The Lancet, 2, 366, 1978.

not to publish my work the outcome might not be so bad. I sat upright, incredulous, then slumped forward with my head in my hands. This couldn't be happening. By then I had multiple staff and the clinic had a fantastic reputation; the HFEA had just started to produce statistics on clinics' success rates and we were the most successful in the country. Simon had only just joined me and was so proud to be Medical Director of the country's number one IVF clinic – how could I let him down? I flew home and took the only action I could at that point, which was to ask the editor of *The Lancet* to pull the case study – I figured if it didn't go public it would be easier for the regulator to go easier on us. 'We can't', the editor said. 'It's gone to print. It was so significant we didn't want to wait.'

As I sat in my office digesting this news, despair turned to fury. 'Who the hell are these people at the HFEA? They'd told me to do what I thought was right for my patient, which was fine when they thought the treatment wouldn't work and no-one would know about it. But now Jenny's pregnant and it's about to hit the medical headlines, they're punishing me and the clinic. Who are they to be the arbiters of how I communicate medical scientific progress with my colleagues and peers? I'm not co-operating with them. I'm just not.' After I calmed down, however, another thought dawned on me which was that my real problem was not the article, it was working out how to protect the livelihoods of my staff and the reputation of Nurture.

Simon and I were summoned to a hearing at the HFEA in London, both of us fearing this would be the perfect opportunity for it to show its teeth by revoking an IVF clinic licence for the first time. Simon barely slept in the run-up and I wasn't much better. There was one trick I had up my sleeve, though, which was a letter I'd written to the HFEA a year beforehand in which I'd disclosed the pioneering work we were doing on male fertility treatment and predicted that soon we might be approached by a man without any mature sperm asking for help, as we had been in Gavin's case. The relevant act of parliament only covers a scenario containing 'a permissible egg and a permissible sperm', and it defines a sperm as 'a male gamete that's capable of undergoing the process of fertilisation'. No-one at the time of the Act had predicted a spermatid could fertilise an egg, but I knew this scenario might arise one day. What was I allowed to do with an immature sperm, such as a spermatid, I asked? The HFEA had never replied to me.

With a flourish I produced this letter in the meeting and wasn't surprised to learn the people interviewing us didn't know anything about it (although the HFEA later admitted the letter had been received). 'I asked you before what would happen if this kind of case were to arise, but you didn't reply.' I said. 'Louise Brown would never have had a chance of being conceived under these conditions.' The result was they rapped our knuckles but kept our licence intact, admonishing us with a warning that we needed to notify them in advance of new developments in future (which of course I'd done). We got away with it but I don't think Simon was ever quite the same again; the experience turned his black mop of hair grey.

The world's first baby conceived from a spermatid, Susan, was born healthy a few months later. Simon and I flew to Aberdeen for the birth, and as he was pictured holding her he said to me, 'I'm pinning your feet to the floor from now on – or one of them at least.' Our paper was published in The Lancet,[13] although the HFEA had effectively banned the procedure from happening again in the UK. Not long afterwards other similar spermatid babies were born worldwide. Susan is a young woman now, and the only child the Os were able to have together because of the ban. Funnily enough, not long ago I was asked by a woman who'd seen my name associated with this case if I could help her and her husband, so I wrote to a senior member of the HFEA to ask if the moratorium had ever been lifted. He told me he had no idea and would get back to me (I've yet to receive a reply).

There are, of course, different sides to this story but the central issue is that of people's lives. I take the libertarian philosophy of not interfering in the decisions of others; if the risks can't be absolutely calculated, who has the right to make choices on behalf of an infertile couple? If this case were to happen today I expect the HFEA would simply say 'no' at the outset. It would defend itself by saying medical research is a different animal to what it was before the regulator existed, and that there must be evidence in advance for everything now.

The gold standard of such evidence is the carrying out of randomised controlled trials before rolling a treatment out;

---

[13] Fishel, Green et al. 1995.

these are designed to prove something is completely safe. There are three main issues with them however. The first is it can be years before they produce definitive answers, and this is too long for couples who are desperate for a baby right now. Currently there's a live trial that's been going for nearly a decade – that's like saying to a woman who wants an abortion it can be done in ten months' time. Next comes the plea for funding, often for millions of pounds or dollars. Who's going to pay for that? And third comes the persuading of hundreds of patients with comparable characteristics to take part, which is fraught with difficulties. Imagine being a woman in your forties and being given the opportunity to either pay for your own treatment or have it for free as part of a trial. You might pick the free option, but there's a catch: you could be randomised into a control group that receives no new treatment, thereby scuppering your chances of having a baby at all. What would you choose?

All IVF scientists would love to carry out proper trials for everything, but you can see why this isn't always possible. I had hoped for a third way, which was to take the wonderful opportunity the NHS affords us for the small percentage of IVF patients it pays for. For instance, if we were to add a new treatment to the conventional IVF process, with the latter being already funded, the money needed for a trial would be far less. It wouldn't cost the NHS or patients anything and would only cost us the research element. But we can't do it because the NHS doesn't allow patients to have additional treatments – what it calls 'top-ups' – even if these are externally funded. That's utterly absurd and restricts research. The paradox is that the only way to prove a technique is safe is to do trials, and trials involve practising the very technique we're not yet allowed to do. I felt so strongly about this I wrote an editorial in one of the scientific journals on this very point.[14]

I wouldn't want you to think my Nurture years were all taken up with world-first cases and battles with the HFEA, though. I spent much of my time treating hundreds of patients, publishing research, and writing books. There was also plenty of travelling, particularly to Italy, Cairo, Greece, and Johannesburg, working with fertility teams who wanted our skills. It wouldn't be an exaggeration to say it was a rollercoaster ride of research

---

[14]   Fishel, 2013.

and patient success highs, interspersed with HFEA lows. However, that ride was about to plunge lower than I'd ever thought possible.

To understand what happened next we have to return to the establishment of Nurture. When I and my team first opened it, I created a clear ethos for the clinic, which was that all the profits would be ploughed back into research, teaching, and training for the ultimate benefit of our patients. Our brochure had the strapline 'non profit-making', with an explanation of what we planned to do with surplus funds clearly emblazoned across it. And profits there certainly were: by the time we'd been open for two or three years, we were clearing at least £750,000 a year.

In 1995, I worked on a joint research project about DNA in sperm imprinting with two colleagues of mine, publishing three papers on it the year after and applying for further funding at the same time.[15] This would cost around £10,000 – a drop in the ocean of Nurture's profits. When the university turned me down I thought they were kidding, but soon I started to wonder where those surpluses were going every year. Malcolm had just been promoted to Dean of the Medical Faculty and had always been supportive of me, so I asked him what to do. He directed me to the university's Vice Chancellor, Colin Campbell. I went to see Campbell and reminded him of Nurture's promise to patients to direct the profits from their fees into research and teaching. Surely after five years of operation these profits should now be sent to the right place? He promised a review of the finances, but eighteen months later I'd still heard nothing. I started making noises about it around the university. 'All I'm asking for is a transparent committee to monitor where the money is going', I said. 'I don't care if the Vice Chancellor, the Dean, and the Head of Department take their cuts, as long as I know the rest is available for Nurture.' My pleas fell on deaf ears.

A while after this I was delighted to be called to Campbell's office; at last he was going to give me the chance to talk about this committee. In retrospect I should never have gone on my own, but I wasn't expecting what I found when I arrived. As I entered the room I was surprised to see the university Bursar sitting beside Campbell. That was odd. Campbell, however,

---

15   Scobie et al. 1996; Aslam and Fishel 1996; Fishel, Aslam et al. 1996.

seemed in an expansive mood and asked me to take a seat. But
as the conversation turned to money he grew more aggressive,
asserting he ran the university and that what happened to the
funds was up to him. At that point he stood up, strode to his
safe, unlocked it, and brought out a thick document.

'You've heard of Lord Irvine, I take it?' I replied I had –
he was Prime Minister Tony Blair's Lord Chancellor, the Head
of the Judiciary, and – as I understood it – someone who was
personally known to Campbell. The Vice Chancellor slammed
the document on the table in front of me. 'I've had none other
than Lord Irvine review your contract, and he confirms I can
dismiss you whenever I like.'

I swallowed hard as I thought of how to reply, but there was
nothing to say. Deciding to rescue whatever dignity I could, I
stood up and walked from the room, and once I reached the
safety of the corridor outside took a deep breath to steady my
nerves. How deluded I'd been. Up until then I'd seen myself as
a blue-eyed boy of the university – the one who was helping
it achieve so many wonderful things and bolster its name
internationally. How arrogant that seemed now, and how
stupid. It was clear to me Campbell wasn't going to do a damn
jot about the research money because it was just a cash cow for
the university.

Walking back to my office from the main campus, I stewed
over how unfair and unnecessary this situation was. Nurture
was going so well. Why not celebrate it instead of exploiting it?
It was decision time. 'Do I put up and shut up', I thought. 'Or
do I walk away?' It was a tough one because I felt I'd created
something special at Nurture and the last thing I wanted was to
upset yet another set of loyal colleagues. And yet staying would
feel so wrong. That night I talked to Judy about it; we decided
me leaving was the only option but that I should wait a while
before I told anyone just to make sure.

Previously I'd worked in South Africa with colleagues using
a new technique called electro-ejaculation, which was a way
of enabling men with spinal cord injuries to ejaculate. I would
use the resulting sperm to fertilise their partners' eggs with
my micro-injection technology. One of the cases there was a
beautiful young couple. The man was a surfer who'd become
paraplegic when he'd flipped a wave and hit the back of his neck.
Desperate to have children, they searched all over the country
only to be told by everyone they consulted it was impossible.

When they discovered this innovation, they were elated. My South African colleague, Dr Lawrence Gobetz, carried out the electro-ejaculation procedure while I did the preparations and sperm injections and created the embryos. We transferred the embryo and they eventually had a wonderful baby. Some nine months later I appeared on a South African TV show on channel M-Net called *Carte Blanche*, a current affairs programme. The episode related the couple's tragedy, but also talked about what we'd done and demonstrated how micro-injection worked. As the credits were about to roll, the surfer was wheeled in by his wife as he held their newborn. It was marvellous.

Shortly after my encounter with Campbell I travelled back to Johannesburg for another run of these spinal cord injury cases. I'd already decided to introduce it to Nurture and had persuaded my colleague and friend Ken Dowell to come with me to learn how to do it. On the flight back Ken and I were sipping our drinks. I couldn't hold it in any longer. 'Ken, I've got something to tell you. You're the first to know and I'm trusting you to keep this quiet, but I can't stay any longer at Nurture. I'm going to resign when we get back.' Ken went quiet for a while, but when he eventually spoke it was only to say, 'Simon, wherever you're going, I'm coming with you.' I couldn't believe it – how comforting that was. In the end he and I did resign together, although looking back on it I can't believe how naive I was to think all I was doing was resigning from a job.

As part of our resignation plans, Ken and I decided we'd approach BMI, the owners of my old clinic at the Park Hospital, to see if they'd be interested in us partnering with them; they agreed to discuss it and seemed positive. Given its proximity to Nurture, only nine miles away, we knew this could be a controversial move so we consulted lawyers at Eversheds before we made any announcements. The advice we were given was under no circumstances to tell anyone about it before we resigned, because otherwise we could be accused of enticing our staff to a competitor – something with serious ramifications. I could see their point, but it was one of the hardest requests ever made of me. Not being able to let my colleagues know in advance what I was planning made me feel deceitful, and ironically, to make matters worse, I was at this time awarded a Professorial Chair called an *ad hominem*. This is a special kind of Chair for life and being nominated for it is secretive process. It's also time consuming as it's adjudicated by several international referees, so it must have been started six months earlier. I had no idea about it until I was told. It was announced in December 1996 and the following February a surprise party was held for me in the department, only a few weeks before I eventually left. It felt horrible to accept this honour when I knew I was going to go, which led to even more soul searching. I almost went back on my decision but Judy and I had just had a baby, Savannah, and I knew I didn't want to be the kind of dad who works in a place that stops him fulfilling his promises to his patients.

When my resignation day finally came only two months later, it was a huge shock to everyone. I'd been awarded a Chair, Nurture was flying – why on earth would I leave? Many of my colleagues were understandably hurt and angry with me for being so secretive. Despite this I felt a rush of relief about being honest, which was probably why I was more open with everyone about my reasons for leaving than was wise. Soon my anger about the research funds being siphoned off became campus news. It wasn't long before our recently appointed Head of Department, Ian Johnson, called me to his office. Again, in my naivety I thought this meeting would be much like when anyone else resigns, because so far he'd been genial about it; I assumed it would be a 'goodbye and good luck' conversation. How wrong I was. I was told I wasn't allowed to work my notice at Nurture and that I must clear out immediately. All I was permitted to take were my coat and wallet, not even my own notebooks or the years of valuable research data from Rome and Bourn Hall; I could collect them at a later date. (Although I asked for them back several times over the following months I never received them.)

The one comfort in all this was that it made me realise how much my colleagues valued me. Some were hurt or bemused, but most told me in one way or another that they'd worked there because of me, and because of what I believed in. Could they come with me, they asked? I couldn't offer them a job for legal reasons, I could only tell them where I was going and when, and that if my new venture needed staff the hospital would advertise for them. When the university later tried to sue me for enticing staff and subpoenaed every single one of them to question them, they were able to put their hands on their hearts and say they had no idea I was leaving before I announced it. Thank goodness for sound legal advice.

This was to be the last time for a while that I could relax around the law. At 5 pm on a Friday night a few weeks later while Judy and I were relaxing at home, a man in a dark suit knocked on the door. 'Are you Simon Fishel?' he said, thrusting an envelope into my hands. 'You've been served with a writ from the University of Nottingham.'

My first thought was, 'What the hell is a writ? I'm a scientist not a lawyer.' My next thought was, 'And how on earth am I going to get any legal help at this time of the week?' (I later learned this is a standard tactic for those who want to make legal issues as nasty as possible – issue a writ on a Friday evening). There was no-one I could call then so I had to wait until Monday before I could get hold of Eversheds, by which time I was almost beside myself with worry. I was met with a soothing response.

'This is just the university beating its chest', they reassured me. 'We'll sort it out, it's contract law. It shouldn't take too long to resolve and you'll only need to set aside £20,000.'

While Eversheds was working on the case I went on a long-planned weekend visit to my mum in Liverpool. On the Saturday evening I received a late-night phone call. 'You don't know me but I'm a journalist for the Mail on Sunday. I recommend you buy it tomorrow.' The phone went dead.

Needless to say, I spent a sleepless night debating with myself about whether I should keep it to myself for now or tell my mum and have her worry too. I decided to wait until I'd seen the paper. First thing on Sunday I went out and bought a copy, opening it with a thudding heart. I couldn't believe my eyes. There in front of me was a large spread, detailing how, in my view, I'd 'stolen the university's crown jewels' and that it was going to sue me. It was truly awful to see this in the national press, especially as I was still technically a member of staff (my contract had not yet terminated). Until the writ, I'd never been given an inkling by any of my superiors that I'd committed any wrongdoing.

It got worse. That evening, Mum and I watched the TV news helplessly as an ITN reporter stood outside the Queens Medical Centre at the university, announcing I was being sued for doing consultation work abroad without the university's knowledge. Even the reporter had to acknowledge this was a bizarre accusation. He held up a university newsletter from the Medical School hailing that very same work – there was nothing secret about it. Unfortunately the BBC correspondent wasn't so neutral, which I was upset about, considering Nurture had given them lots of material over the years for their programmes about IVF. I couldn't believe what I was seeing and hearing and could only imagine what my colleagues at home and abroad were thinking about me. It was as bad as it gets. It was shocking.

The following week I got in touch with Stephen Collier, the lawyer who'd signed me to the Park Hospital back in 1985. He was now on the board of its owners, BMI, as their legal counsel. Clearly this media storm, only a month after my resignation and two months before I could start another job, would dislodge my offer from them. But Stephen said not to worry. He did some digging and came to the conclusion that all the university wanted at that point was to stop me and Ken moving to the Park Hospital. He also told me that as a member of staff at the university (which I still technically was) it was incumbent on my employer to give me a warning if it felt I'd committed a misdemeanour, not to issue me with a writ. I assured Stephen I'd gained permission for me and my colleagues to work abroad and had been completely open about it. 'Let's hit the pause button on the move for now', he suggested. 'It'll give the university a chance to cool down and forestall any negative publicity for the hospital.'

There was no choice but to carry on with my work plans, and after some time Stephen was able to assure me that my agreement with BMI would be honoured come what may. So Ken and I could go ahead with our plan to partner up with the Park IVF Clinic, and on 4 August 1997, the documents were signed. We bought out 50 per cent of the clinic using funds we'd borrowed from BMI – it took all we could afford. We also decided to give it a new name: the Centre for Assisted Reproduction, or CARE. My erstwhile colleague John Webster was hugely magnanimous about my return, given I'd abandoned him there when I'd left before. Actually the Park clinic was dying by then because we'd been so successful at Nurture; when I'd departed it was carrying out 1,300 cycles a year and now it was down to 250. We believed in this venture, and shortly afterwards the Park Hospital advertised for staff. Three immediately joined us, of whom two are still with me after all these years: Wanda and Judith. Eventually many others applied too, including my three best embryologists, two of whom remain at CARE today. One of them was Alison Campbell, who is now Director of Embryology for CARE; she'd joined me in 1992 on the Master's degree course in its first year, and because she was late applying they originally wouldn't take her. I fought for her and she turned out to be one of the best embryologists on the planet. In all, seventeen staff from Nurture made their way to the Park clinic. It makes me feel terrible to think all these good people were later brought into a court room to be grilled under oath.

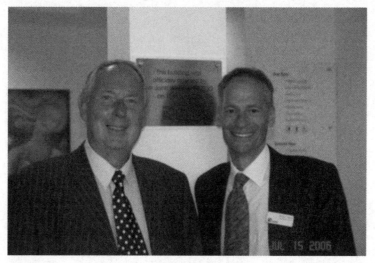

Figure 5.2: John Webster and me at the opening of John Webster House, CARE, 2016

There was a sting in the tail to this successful start. The exodus of experienced staff decimated Nurture and caused Campbell to ramp his legal action up a gear. For him, it was now personal. Malcolm, my boss at the university and until then a good friend, said to me Campbell had told him: 'Malcolm, it doesn't really matter what goes in the affidavit for the lawyers. Fishel will never see court.' Of course, I could see why Campbell would feel riled about the establishment of CARE but I never thought he would become as aggressive as he did. Things were about to get bad. Very bad.

Chapter 6
Bankruptcy Looms
1997–2001

Establishing the extent and nature of the university's claims against me took lawyers on both sides several months, with the end result being a staggeringly long list of twenty-one accusations. There were two that were more important than the rest. The first was the claim that because my job title at Nurture had been Scientific Director, I was considered a fiduciary (a word I'd never heard before) and any consultation work abroad I'd carried out while working there belonged to the university rather than me. According to Campbell, I should therefore pay the university the overblown sum of £400,000 – an amount that would bankrupt me on its own, let alone with added legal costs. My counter-argument was that it was customary for academics to carry out consultancy work on their own account, and that at many universities there were people with the word 'Director' in their job title without it being treated as the equivalent of a board director in a commercial company. The second was that I'd breached my contract by not gaining the proper permission to work outside the university and Nurture. In fact I'd received permission both from my department and from the Dean of the Medical School, which was common practice in universities.

The cornerstone of the university's case against me, therefore, was that I'd hidden my foreign work in order to exploit it for my own benefit. This came as a huge shock to me and others, because the university had been so proud of Nurture's international accomplishments it had even promoted them in its newsletter; there was no way it didn't know what I was doing abroad. Ironically, the research and treatments I undertook in various foreign countries had kept Nurture at the cutting edge of IVF and helped it attract patients from all over the world. What's more, they enabled me to bring in top rate staff who were delighted to be part of something exceptional, and students who applied to the Master's degree course on the basis of our world-leading techniques.

After this there were a further nineteen claims, some of them bizarre, including accusations I had clandestine bank accounts and a secret car hidden somewhere. Apparently I'd been doing all sorts of things! At this stage it all looked so ridiculous I was fairly sure it would be cleared up without any serious problems, but it was still a weight on my shoulders. And my £20,000 with Eversheds didn't last long because I had to go through a series of court hearings to establish the exact nature of the case.

This was when my first serious setback occurred. Over the years the university had cleverly ensured it used all the lawyers in town; this meant if any law firm were to act against the university it could have a conflict of interest. After a few months the university discovered that in the dim and distant past Eversheds had acted for it and made a fuss about its work with me, and clearly this was now extending way beyond simple contract law. That, together with its desire not to annoy a large institution in a relatively small town, led it to resign my case. Imagine being told by a big-name law firm that your case is much more complex than it first thought, and it could no longer defend me – this was a serious blow to my confidence.

As I was sitting at home one day wondering what on earth to do next I received a phone call from one of my cousins, who ran a successful business. 'Si, how are things going?' he asked. 'I've been reading about your case in the papers.' I told him I was at a loss as to what to do, because not only did I have a legal action running against me, my lawyers had deserted me too. 'Don't worry', he said. 'Let's see if I can help you out. I'll ask our cousin Joe to take on your case and my company will underwrite the costs. What else are families for?'

Joe, the man he was referring to, was a lawyer in our family and the fact that the two of them were prepared to help me for no charge was indescribably uplifting. Joe suggested I come down to see him at his office, and while we were discussing the claims against me the phone rang. It was my wife Judy.

'I'm calling from a neighbour's – our phone's been cut off. When I spoke to the phone company they told me we'd said we were moving, and to cancel our account.'

As I related this to Joe, a worried look crossed his face and he immediately asked to speak to Judy. 'Go outside and take a look at your bins', he said.

'Bins?' I asked. 'What are you talking about?'

'I know what goes on in these cases', he replied. 'They try to rattle the plaintiff by doing things like this to unsettle them. Not only have they got your phone cut off, they'll also be rooting through your bins at night trying to find dirt on you and see if you're disposing of any evidence. That's probably how they got hold of enough personal details to impersonate you to the phone company.'

When I realised how far the university would go to put the frighteners on me, I remembered an incident from before I left Nurture. Judy and I had been on a family holiday in Pembrokeshire; we didn't often get the chance to go away so this was precious time together with our children. While we were there I checked my bank account and discovered I hadn't been paid; it was a sizeable sum as it included a bonus I was owed. Because of the terrible mobile reception I had to race around to find a piece of high enough ground to call the university while holding my phone above my head (I probably looked pretty hilarious), and because I couldn't find out what had happened we had to cut short our holiday and return home. A series of arguments with the Bursar ensued, in which I was told it was an administrative error and was finally paid. I got the impression, though, that it was part of a series of attempts to demoralise me so I'd give up my campaign for Nurture's profits to be spent on research.

We finally got our home phone line reinstated, but Joe said this showed a strong letter to the university was needed. He wrote to tell Campbell he could do his worst, but that his client had unlimited funds and would see him all the way to court (of course, to Campbell this was like a red rag to a bull). After this initial letter Joe got to work on my behalf, obtaining witness statements from everyone who was on my side.

The legal wheels rumbled on for a further year, after which I received another phone call from my cousin, this time a less welcome one. He explained Joe had told him he couldn't manage the workload anymore and that it was becoming too complex for him. Given I was starting to sink under the weight of the legalities myself, I understood how he felt and thanked them both for what they'd done. This meant, however, I was back to square one.

A couple of weeks later I was invited to the christening of a patient's baby by her father George, who'd originally come to me for IVF because of the research I'd been pioneering overseas. If I'm honest I didn't much feel like going – the thought of having to put on a smile when all I could think about was what I'd do when I went bankrupt didn't appeal. Thank goodness I did, though, because I can't believe how different my future would have been if I'd stayed at home. After the other guests had gone, George and I poured ourselves a drink and sat outside. He told me he'd been following my story in the press and asked how I was coping. I explained the latest development with Joe. 'I don't think I can carry on anymore', I said. 'I'm considering declaring myself bankrupt – at least that way it will all be over. It just seems there's no other way out.' George looked concerned.

'Look, I know what you've been doing in IVF and I can't believe this case is anything but vindictive. I've got a friend, Patrick, who's a specialist lawyer in this area. Would it be okay if I spoke with him?' he asked. I thanked him but said I had no funds available; he told me not to worry for now and that we'd have a chat after Patrick had had a look at the legal documents so far.

It took some time for Joe to send the files to Patrick as by that stage Joe and I weren't on the best of terms, but eventually they arrived and a few weeks later Patrick invited me over to his house. As I walked in I saw him sitting at his home office desk, frowning.

'I'm glad to be able to help you after everything George has told me about you, Simon', he said. 'But how come you've missed all these court hearings? This is deadly serious – you're aggravating the judicial system. Soon the courts will be so annoyed you'll be lucky if the case doesn't go against you automatically.'

I was aghast. 'What do you mean, missed hearings?'

It transpired Joe hadn't told me about a series of hearings I was supposed to have attended in court, the missing of which could land me in deep trouble. Patrick told me the courts didn't care whether it was my fault or my lawyer's – I was responsible and would pay the price.

Looking up at Patrick, I asked him what I should do next. 'We have a massive amount of work to do', he said. 'First I'll have to grovel to the courts because of your missing hearings. They won't like you for doing that and then changing lawyers – they'll think you're up to no good. But I'll try to convince them it wasn't your fault and get the case back on track.'

I was overwhelmed and reiterated I couldn't afford to pay him. 'That's okay', he replied. 'George has agreed to cover your costs in gratitude for what you've done for his family.'

This was almost too magnanimous to comprehend; it was like I had a guardian angel descending from heaven. Patrick spent the next few weeks in urgent negotiations with the courts, explaining why we needed a hearing to discuss why I hadn't been at the other hearings.

It was a hugely pressured time made bearable only by Patrick's unflagging energy and commitment, which was amazing and still seems unbelievable to me. The affidavit he eventually drew up was a huge 250 pages long. Every word was typed by him, all of it in his own time. Sometimes we'd sit together all night; he'd fire a question at me and I'd answer it, dozing off in between times to the sound of his clacking keyboard. And because of George's generosity he never charged me a penny. This was an enormous help as my main worry, apart from clearing my name, was going bankrupt and consequently losing my directorship of CARE, not to mention my four young children who I had to provide for. We'd launched the CARE clinic in Nottingham in 1997, with further ones in Manchester and Sheffield following in 1999 and 2000. It was still a fledgling business, and while I was attending court hearings and working on the affidavit with Patrick, I was also its Managing Director and working regularly until the small hours – sometimes all night. If George and Patrick hadn't helped me the way they did I don't know what I'd have done.

As I mentioned before, the writ contained twenty-one counts against me for a wide variety of supposed misdemeanours. Some of them appeared to come from nowhere. For instance, they claimed I had a secret bank account abroad and that I'd hidden away an expensive car in a bid to reduce my visible assets. It was puzzling why they would make these things up, and where they'd got their evidence from. This was soon to become clear.

In any litigation there's a process called 'discovery', which effectively means spending a day with your lawyer in a room stacked floor to ceiling with boxes of the plaintiff's proof against you. The idea is to go through the boxes with a fine-tooth comb so you can see what they've got before you go to court, and what we discovered was unbelievable.

Shortly before I'd left the university I'd had a Psion handheld computer; if you're old enough to remember them you'll know it was a glorified electronic diary with limited computing functionality. I'd bought it myself and had my whole life on it – contact details for friends, family and colleagues, personal appointments, and so on. When it stopped working I'd taken it to Jessops department store in Nottingham to be fixed along with Judy's, as both were broken. After my resignation I realised I'd not heard from the store so I phoned to ask when they would be ready. They put me on hold while they looked for them and eventually said I'd already collected them. I replied this wasn't possible. 'Come on down and we'll show you', they said. So I went and there, on a signed collection docket for our Psions, was the name of a woman I'd appointed as the administrator for Nurture. It turned out the store had called my university office number and left a message to say they were ready, which had been picked up by her; she'd then handed them over to the university. So our personal property was in the university's hands, enabling it to rifle through our details and pick out anything it could make look suspicious. When I asked for the devices to be returned she gave back Judy's but refused to return mine, claiming it belonged to the institution.

The Psion provided the basis of some of the claims against me, a couple of which were actually quite funny. The clandestine bank account name turned out to be that of our babysitter, and the 'account number' was her phone number. As for the luxury car I'd apparently secreted away, the university claimed it had the registration number D1 SCO. In fact I'd contacted the DVLA (the details of which were on my Psion), to ask if this registration was available when I'd developed the sperm injection technique I'd called DISCO (Direct Injection of the Sperm into the Cytoplasm of the Oocyte). I never went ahead with the registration number, but from this the university manufactured the claim I had a secret car.

There was more. One of the university's more fanciful claims was that Ken Dowell and I had a secret clinic in Dubai, which I was supposedly hiding because I didn't want to disclose the extent of my foreign trips. It even detailed the dates we'd visited, despite the fact I'd never been there in my life. In our discovery session we unearthed Ken's diary at the bottom of one of the countless boxes – it was almost as if they didn't want us to find it. In that diary was a record of every trip Ken had made to his sister, who happened to live in Dubai; clearly the university had extrapolated from this that I'd made a series of lucrative visits there myself. When I mentioned this to Ken he said, 'Do you know, that's amazing because not long ago I came back to my office from theatre and exchanged my white coat for my jacket. In my jacket I found my diary to be missing. I couldn't explain it because my office had been locked and there was no sign of a break-in.'

After I had the day with Patrick going through the boxes, he carried on working on my case. One day he called me up. 'You need to come to my office right now', he said. 'You'll never believe what I've been sent.' I leapt into my car and drove the 100 miles to his office, where I found him with his head poking out over a pile of books and papers. He jumped up in triumph, waving a sheaf of papers. 'Look at this', he said. 'We've got somebody bang to rights. It's a massive data breach, and this kind of information doesn't come cheap. We're going straight to the Data Protection Commissioner with this – it's the kind of thing they're always looking for.' The documents he was brandishing were ones he was sure that whoever was responsible for them would never have wanted leaked, and to this day I don't know how they were obtained and who sent them to him. They included every detail of my bank accounts, even transactions such as my wife's payment for a pair of shoes from a catalogue, my utility bills, and other information even I wasn't aware of. According to the report detailing the transactions, 'Discreet enquiries were undertaken with regard to Banking Facilities of Centres for Assisted Reproduction.' And it went on to say, 'Our agents advise that your subject has never been made bankrupt and as such confidential enquiries were made with the Inland Revenue to establish the current level of income received by your subject.' Together with this was a communication from the private investigator who'd obviously been instructed to dig up the information, and near the end was a telling line: 'With regard to Johannesburg PO, Banco Nazionale Del Lavoro, Rome and Credit Suisse, unfortunately we are unable to locate any further foreign accounts information within the budget available.' Patrick was right, we'd got the university bang to rights.

After the plundering of my Psion and Ken's diary I thought I'd seen every kind of dirty trick, but this left me beyond words. Patrick explained anyone with vast sums of money could infiltrate my personal data in this nefarious way. It didn't help me, though; I still had to defend myself against the claims. When a party can say whatever it likes about someone else, however ridiculous, the recipient still has to go through the tortuous process of defending themselves. I called it civilised violence.

Patrick and I discussed what to do next, and he suggested I should talk to my local MP. 'There's only one problem with that idea', I said. 'He's a long-time buddy of Campbell's, Kenneth Clarke. Having a conversation about this with Clarke isn't going to be easy.' As an alternative I went to see another MP called Alan Simpson, but although it turned out he held the same view of Campbell as I did, he said he was unable to help due to the MPs' code of conduct. So I visited Kenneth Clarke, who greeted me amiably and asked how he could help. This was when I showed him my dossier of the dirty tricks, and questioned if public funds could have been used to breach the Data Protection Act. Clarke looked surprised and said he would look into it, although I never heard anything from him. Something I'll say for Alan Simpson, though, was he wrote several letters to the university after my trial, asking how much it had spent on the action and whether or not the funds had come from Nurture's profits. According to the replies, this question was far too difficult for the university to answer given the huge budgets it controlled.

Many months after my meeting with Clarke, Patrick still hadn't been able to get anywhere with the Department of Public Prosecutions regarding the data breach. One day I went to see him and found him looking shaken. 'I've had a man in a grey suit visit me from the DPC office. They've dropped their investigation into the report and have said there are no fingerprints to link it anywhere.' Patrick had assumed, given the privacy laws had been so blatantly breached, there would be a chance of prosecuting the offender. It was strange the DPC never took it any further.

***

Three years after I'd been served the writ it was finally the morning for the case to go to trial. I awoke with a grey, exhausted shadow in my head. Despite this being the day I'd worked towards for so long, and my chance to show I'd not done anything wrong, it took me a while to drag myself out of bed. What if Campbell had some trick up his sleeve I wasn't aware of? What if the judge didn't believe me? What if I just couldn't get myself through it all? I lay there contemplating the worst. Gradually, though, anger began to crowd out the despair. What right did the university have to hound me like this? If they thought I'd done something wrong while I was working for them, all they had to do was talk to me at the time. Instead they'd trumped up a preposterous series of twenty-one charges against me, all of which I was determined to prove wrong. Thanks to Patrick I would have my day in court.

The trial didn't get off to a promising start because as soon as it had been convened the judge, Patrick Elias, had to declare a conflict of interest: his brother had been a close colleague of Campbell's. The court was adjourned for me to decide if I would allow him to carry on, which I was naturally reluctant to do. 'No way do I want anyone associated with Campbell to be the judge', I said to Patrick. However, Patrick explained from a judicial viewpoint this would be seen as me questioning Elias' impartiality − a big no-no. The next judge to be appointed would then know what I'd accused his predecessor of and could be prejudiced against me. I got the message. The trial started the next day, with Elias presiding.

What followed was three exhausting weeks in the High Court of Justice, with me in the witness stand for two full days. I remember towards the end of my testimony I was asked a question I can no longer recall, but it was based on whether I would do a certain thing again. I replied I would. At that point a little voice in my head piped up: 'That's the wrong answer, Simon.' I glanced at Patrick who was frowning so I said, 'Your honour, can I change my reply? I meant to say "no" your honour, absolutely not.' Afterwards when I had a chance to catch up with Patrick he said to me quietly, 'That's what we lawyers call a "selling your mother" moment. When a witness is exhausted after hours or days on the stand, they no longer know what they're saying. If the judge had asked if you would you sell your own mother, you'd probably have said yes.'

When Campbell was called to the stand my barrister asked him about the time when the university had withheld my salary while I was on holiday in Pembrokeshire. The evidence given by the Bursar, and other university staff who'd actioned the stoppage, indicated Campbell had told them to lie and say it was a clerical error whereas it was in fact an attempt by him to intimidate me. When Campbell was pressed on this event he said (and this is from the court transcript):

> *My barrister*: Let us see if we can call a spade a spade. Was it a lie, in your terminology?
>
> *Campbell*: It was misleading.
>
> *My barrister*: It was misleading. Was it a lie?
>
> *Campbell*: I don't know what [the Bursar] actually said to him. It may have been a small lie.
>
> *My barrister*: Let me read [the Bursar's evidence] again. 'I informed the Vice Chancellor [...] of my decision. As I recall, the Vice Chancellor requested that the delay in payment be notified to Dr Fishel as inefficiency in the University's administrative processes so as to avoid any contractual dispute.' Was it a lie?
>
> *Campbell*: I think it was probably a small lie, yes.
>
> *My barrister*: Only a small lie.

It would be funny if it wasn't so awful. It was, in fact, a clear lie. Through the discovery process, emails had come to light between the Bursar and the Head of HR discussing how I'd asked them why I'd not been paid. Campbell had told them to 'let him sweat'. His aim was to twist my arm behind my back to weaken my negotiating position with him regarding the profits from Nurture that weren't going where I wanted them.

There was also a moment in the trial when the name of a fellow academic called Marcus Filshie was mentioned. He worked at the university and held a directorship of a company that made clips for sterilising fallopian tubes: the 'Filshie clip'. He'd made some money from this legitimate business while working as a lecturer and researcher at the university, just like me. Campbell was asked if he'd expressed as much interest in

Filshie's earnings and his approval status for working outside the university as he had in mine. He seemed unsure what to say.

My barrister: Have you interested yourself in that issue?

Campbell: No. I was told he has resigned from the University.

There was a gasp all round as we looked at each other: Filshie had certainly not resigned from the university – he was very much still there.

The only thing that got me through the trial was the support of my family, Patrick, and some of my colleagues both in Nottingham and from abroad. One of those fellow professionals, Franco Lisi in Italy, was questioned in court by video link. When the judge asked him if I'd traded off the Nurture name to build my reputation in Italy, and if Lisi had wanted to work with me because of Nurture's reputation, he asserted there was no Nurture without me and that no-one in Italy or elsewhere in our field had even heard of Nottingham University except through my work. That was a great moment and a turning point for the judge, because one of the claims against me had been that I'd used Nurture abroad for my own benefit. Someone else who helped was Robert Winston, who gave evidence that the kind of consultancy work I'd been doing was normal for academics. This gave a peer's weight to my case, for which I was grateful, and similar support came from colleagues in Egypt, South Africa, and elsewhere.

After the trial was over I felt hugely relieved, but we still had to wait several weeks for the verdict on 19 January 2000. When it came it was better than I expected, although I was still disappointed the judge wasn't harsher on the university. It was one of those situations in which both sides claim a victory (in Patrick's words, it went to penalties). Of the list of claims against me, I won nineteen and lost only two. I was particularly pleased when judge Elias gave this view of me: 'Although he wanted to capitalise on his skills, he is not in my view a man who is driven by the desire to maximise income at all cost [...] Mammon can be an insidious subverter. However, on the evidence before me, the university has not satisfied me that Dr Fishel did in fact succumb to that deception.'[16] In other words

---

[16]   Nottingham University v Fishel (2000) IRLR 471, HC.

he saw I was someone who wasn't motivated purely by money, and that meant a lot.

Legally speaking, my main triumph was I was found not to be a fiduciary so I didn't have to account to the university for my foreign fees. Where I lost was in that I was found to have been in technical breach of my contract by not gaining the proper permission to do the work abroad. My legal terms said I needed to receive permission from the Senate to carry out work outside the university; in reality nobody in my position ever did this because the Head of the Department's agreement was considered enough. This was a blow but the judge's conclusion was a comfort because it acknowledged this had caused no harm to the university. 'I find that Dr Fishel is liable for breach of contract, but since I have found that there is no loss to the university, there are no damages.'[17]

I was also pleased to be exonerated of having carried out this work without the university's knowledge. Judge Elias had this to say about it: 'It is clear beyond doubt that Professors Symonds and Johnson were aware that consultancy work was being done abroad by Dr Fishel. Indeed, they positively encouraged it.' I was happy to see the truth come to light, because I'd said all along it was wrong to imply that I had done it in secret.

At this point the judge asked both parties to return to court for the awarding of costs. I knew this would be the moment when we'd discover who'd really won so I looked forward to it, but we had to wait a year because the university kept prevaricating. Before the big day, though, an unexpected event occurred: Patrick received a letter from the university offering to settle the case with immediate effect. The sting in the tail was I would have to sign a confidentiality agreement, meaning I could not discuss its terms. Patrick didn't know why the university had suddenly changed tack but urged me to accept the offer.

So we did, and in March 2001 it was all over. And guess what – a week later it was announced Campbell was to be Her Majesty's First Commissioner of Judicial Appointments, serving under his friend Derry Irvine. I assumed from the urgent change in the university's position that it needed to conclude the case with me promptly, so he could be appointed to the role

---

[17]   Ibid.

without it hanging over him. I have to hand it to Campbell – he never missed an opportunity. Before he resigned from the university in 2008 he acquired a well-documented 90% salary rise, bringing him income and benefits of over £550,000 a year (the average vice chancellor's salary at the time was £190,000).[18] Given pensions were still based on final salary then, it's not a stretch to conclude he was the better off for it.

Professor Alan Prichard, Pro Vice Chancellor and Head of Law at Nottingham University, wrote an interesting precis of the case. He said the judge found I had broken my contract, but:

> the university had not only suffered no loss, but had actually derived substantial benefit from the breach. Needless to say, such a finding renders the university's pursuit of the issue at great cost to public funds utterly unjustifiable when it could have been dealt with amicably. The judge also upheld Dr Fishel's integrity and good faith on all issues, even on the one he lost over. That makes the sustained assault on his honesty and standing all the more deplorable – especially since Dr Fishel twice in September 1998 offered the university a settlement that would have given it much more than what it can now achieve under the judgment. (Unpublished appraisal of judgment, Alan Prichard)

You may wonder why I'm writing about all this now. The answer is, even though nearly twenty years have gone by and I've been able to get most of it into perspective, the more I think about it the more amazing it seems. Judge Elias' judgment even spawned what became known as the 'Fishel effect' in law, which defines the financial parameters for university employees doing consultancy work.

You might also have found yourself imagining what it must have been like for me and my family during those three years of legal hell. When I look back on it my primary memory is of extreme tiredness and prolonged periods of duress. I had

---

[18] www.ucu.org.uk/article/3769/Uni-bosses-pay-on-a-par-with-the-prime-minister-after-huge-rises?list=3656. www.theguardian.com/education/2009/mar/19/administration-universityfunding.

four children to support, the youngest of whom was born just a few months before I received the writ. I also felt enormously hurt by the reactions of some of my colleagues. Many of them had come to my wedding to my second wife Judy; we'd had an intimate reception with only thirty people, of whom a third were from Nurture and the university, as Judy worked at Nurture too. After I left, the majority of the university staff – but thankfully not my Nurture colleagues – did the university's bidding by going against me in some way. This made looking back on the wedding photos pretty upsetting for a long time. I remember coming home one day shortly after the writ to find Judy in distress because an IT manager from the university had knocked on the door while I'd been out and demanded she hand over my university computer, which had a lot of private information on. He'd been a good friend until then.

In October 2000, well after I had left, I was a passenger in the Hatfield train crash which killed four people and injured more than seventy. Luckily I survived with only a few hairline cracked bones and emotional bruises, although I was in a carriage that had flipped over, but was recently told that a professor at Nottingham in the same department as me had said at the time, 'It's a pity Fishel didn't die in that crash.' The colleague who relayed this to me said she was so shocked by the comment she decided to leave. I often asked myself what all those years with some of those people had counted for.

In my darkest days, a few months before the trial, I did doubt if I could carry on. I don't think I'd have done anything drastic because that would have been the coward's way out, especially when I had my family to look after. I also remember coming home late one night and turning on the TV to relax. The programme that came on was about the work of Simon Wiesenthal, the courageous and persistent man who became known as the 'Nazi Hunter'. I watched it to the end. If he could keep going in the face of what he had to deal with, so could I. And when I considered the suffering of the people who perished or survived the Holocaust, it was obvious my own troubles were nothing in comparison. That was the moment when I realised if I lost my health or integrity, the university would win. If I could keep those two things intact, in time there was no reason why I couldn't gain everything else back. It was a turning point and enabled me to keep going.

Having said that, maybe it was also a growing-up time, battering out the last vestiges of my naivety. When I was interviewed for a personal profile by the *European Journal of Andrology* some time afterwards, and the journalist asked me what my worst professional mistake had been, and I said it was believing certain senior academics would be honourable men. I didn't believe they'd publish it, but they did. The trial also taught me how easily brilliant things can be destroyed. All I'd wanted was for the university to allocate Nurture's profits the way it had initially agreed and to have some transparency around it, and yet somehow this had set in motion a series of catastrophic events that finished off the clinic and almost me as well.

Another thing I learned was that there are friends, and there are true friends. George, my guardian angel, not only saved my life on a practical level but, together with Patrick, he gave me back my self-respect and professional life because he stopped me from going bankrupt. What's more, prior to the case I'd been an inspector for the HFEA, but it suspended me for the period of the writ and for some time after the trial. A family friend, Charles, sent the HFEA a transcript of the judgment and suggested it revisit the suspension; the HFEA decided I no longer had a case to answer and re-established me at once. There was Alan Prichard, who didn't know me at all but gave me constant solace through his advice, time, energy and support. He wrote to me nearly every week, which was incredibly generous of him given his high standing at the university; he had much to lose. Also John Webster, who was a steadfast support throughout. And I can't forget my loyal colleagues at CARE who'd given up their jobs at Nurture to follow me. Finally there was Stephen Collier the barrister and counsel to the board of BMI. Although he had commercial interests at BMI to worry about, he signed the augmentation of the CARE venture with me and Ken in August 1997, only months after the media controversy initiated by the university. He even helped me store my huge collection of lever arch files in his garage before transferring them to the Royal Courts of Justice when the trial began.

So the legal action was a defining moment in my life and career, but I was as aware then as I am now, that it was nothing to do with IVF. It was time to begin the next phase of my work as Scientific and Managing Director of CARE, the organisation that was to become the UK's largest and most successful chain of IVF clinics.

Chapter 7

CARE: The Battle for Miracles Continues

1997–Present

Although my early years as Scientific Director of CARE were scarred by the legal action with the university, in every other way they were a wonderful time of growth and learning. Ken Dowell and I had bought a 50 per cent share of the Park Hospital clinic in Nottingham between us, and re-named it CARE. To my delight and relief, my long-time colleague and friend John Webster agreed to stay on as Medical Director and we quickly put in place an excellent team of people, most of whom came from Nurture.

That was the good news. The bad news was that in its previous guise as the Park Clinic, the unit's work had been decimated by the success we'd generated nine miles up the road at Nurture, and was only carrying out around 250 cycles of IVF a year. There was much peddling to do to establish CARE's reputation as the place to go for assisted conception in the area, with no obvious way to achieve it. I needed divine intervention, and fast.

Miraculously, as miracles do, it arrived in the form of a dusty collection of folders. I came across them in a drawer at the clinic – they'd clearly been tucked away since the Park days – and on closer inspection they turned out to be an enormous bunch of patient files for women who required egg donation. When I asked the administration staff what the records were doing there, I was told they'd been abandoned because 'we don't really do egg donation here anymore'. This was our opportunity! John and I had carried out the UK's first IVF with a donated egg back in 1986 for Susan Ooi, who'd had eggs donated from her sister, so we knew how to carry out this complex procedure.

'We're crazy if we don't do something with this', I said. 'Here's a group of patients who need our help, and they're ready and waiting for us.' I took the notes home with me that night and started calling the women one by one, asking if they still wanted a donor egg. It took me and my wife Judy weeks to get hold of them all and most said they were desperate for help.

Our next task was to rapidly build up a bank of egg donors for these recipients. Judy was working at the clinic part-time now that our daughter Savannah was a year old. She had a nursing background and had also owned her own PR company in the past, so was the ideal person to take charge of the project. She appeared on all the local radio stations asking women to donate and set up a system called Egg Share Donation, in which women with healthy eggs could give theirs in exchange for lower cost IVF treatment. The response was incredible – our phones rang constantly with women asking if they could donate. This was all the more amazing given the concept of egg donation wasn't well known at the time.

Over the next couple of years, Judy, my colleague Simon Thornton, and I turned our egg donation programme into the biggest in the country, and by the time it was flying we were carrying out an unprecedented fifteen to twenty donor egg IVF cases a month. What made it all the more satisfying was that, because some of it gave us access to donor eggs from younger women with no fertility problems, this boosted our results. This programme was pivotal in enabling us to survive the first year or two of being open as a clinic, and even today CARE is still the largest donated egg provider in the UK. We eventually built up a surrogacy programme to accompany it, with our Manchester clinic being the largest provider of surrogacy implantations in the country.

Of course there were, and still are, ethical and practical issues concerning the use of donated eggs. Because egg donors had to be anonymous by law, and because the technology in those days limited us only to fresh egg donation, we had to set up a complex procedure to synchronise the collection of the egg, the fertilisation of the embryo, and its implantation. This entailed the programming of two women's cycles to run concurrently: one to collect the eggs and the other to prepare the womb to receive them. Can you imagine how tricky it was to make sure the donor and recipient didn't accidentally bump into one another in reception? A breach of confidentiality would have lost us our licence. Thankfully we're now able to freeze eggs for storing in our egg bank which makes the practicalities far simpler.

Times have moved on, however, with two major shifts having had an impact on egg donation today. The first is that the HFEA agreed donors could be paid a nominal sum, which has made recruitment easier. But the more important change is that in 2005 it decided, almost overnight and in a complete about-turn, to institute a national registry for donors. Since then all children born from a donated egg can ask to see the donor's details when they turn eighteen. In the short term this almost extinguished women's willingness to donate eggs, with the result that couples started going abroad. It's now slowly built back up but we still reckon around 7,000 couples a year travel to foreign countries from the UK. You can't stop people doing what they want, but we'd rather they did it here where it's safe and regulated.

I believe there should be no family secrets about egg and sperm donation, and the earlier the child is told the better they're able to deal with it. There are now helpful and sensitive books which guide parents on introducing the topic to their children. Because today, more than ever, no donation is untraceable, especially now that we have access to so much genetic information about ourselves. A child may find out in their biology lesson at school, for instance, that they're a different blood group to their parents, or visit one of the family tree tracing websites and discover their genes are incompatible (these sites can map your child's genetic origins). It's better the child should know from its parents than to find out by surprise or have to go behind their backs. However, despite our best

efforts, we still find many couples don't want to be open with
their children so they go abroad to make it anonymous.

***

Because setting up the clinic and coping with my legal problems
took up all my time at the beginning of CARE, I certainly wasn't
on the look-out for any exciting cases. In fact, although you
may find this hard to believe, I rarely am – they just seem to
find their way to me regardless. It was like this when I was
invited to take part in a TV chat show in Leeds; little did I know
it would prepare the ground for an encounter that would land
my activities in court.

   As I was sitting in the green room after the show I got
chatting to some of the other guests. One of them was a
policeman who'd become a woman and the other two were
a couple called Shahana and Raj Hashmi. Shahana was quiet
and dignified and I'd admired her courage when she'd talked
on the programme about her two-year-old son Zain, who had
beta thalassaemia. This is a genetic blood disorder that prevents
a child from metabolising oxygen properly, leaving them
on a cocktail of drugs and blood transfusions for the rest of
their dramatically shortened life. It can be cured by stem cell
donation but it has to be the perfect match from the donor for it
to work. Shahana and her husband had four other children but
none was a match for Zain. While we were sitting in that green
room I noticed her go quiet, as if she was deeply considering
something. Then she turned to me. 'You're the IVF doctor,
aren't you?' she asked. I replied that I was. 'I'm looking for a
way of curing Zain. If we could have a baby who was a match we
could take stem cells from the baby's placenta and give them to
Zain. We'd love another child anyway, but we want to make sure
Zain can be cured too. The only problem is, the hospital have
told us it's not possible. Can you help?'

   My heart went out to her because I knew IVF was Zain's
only hope. The Hashmis had scoured the donor banks in vain
to find an exact donor match, so what were their options?
Keep rolling the reproductive dice in the hope of having
another baby who happened to be a match? Imagine having
more children with the disease, or who weren't a match. It
was cruel position to be in. Their chance of having a baby
naturally who was both disease-free and a match was only

three in sixteen, so even embryo selection wasn't a sure bet. But at least it would mean they didn't need to risk having more babies with beta thalassaemia. 'It's medically possible to create embryos and select one that's a match', I told her. 'But embryo selection for the purpose of helping a sibling, rather than for the baby itself, is not allowed in the UK. Given your situation this seems a crazy rule to me, so let me see if I can find out any more for you.'

I got on the phone with some colleagues in the US and asked if they'd be willing to help. There was a technology just developed called Pre-Implantation Genetic Diagnosis, or PGD, which is now available all over the world. We were already using it to a certain extent to screen embryos for familial genetic conditions, thereby enabling us to select the embryos that were free of disease; this was permissible under UK law at the time. However, we couldn't screen embryos with the aim of helping a sibling, which could only be done in the US. I suggested to Shahana we create the embryos here, take biopsies from them for screening in the US, and if this showed a match the couple could travel to the US to have them implanted. Or we could fight to get the process accepted here. She said she'd be willing to take on the challenge.

Time was against us as Shahana was in her late thirties, producing fewer eggs as the months went by. Lengthy conversations with the US dragged things out but were as nothing compared to the hoops we had to jump through with the HFEA. The creation of a 'saviour sibling', as it became known, had never been attempted in the UK before so I had to throw all my persuasive efforts into it. First it went through our own ethical committee, which supported the endeavour; this was absolutely essential before we could even think of approaching the regulator. As Shahana commented to the media at the time, '[Zain] will die if the HFEA decision is negative. We will go to the end of the world to get what we feel is right for Zain. This new baby will be very special because, hopefully, he'll be a match and save his brother.'[19] Simultaneously I had to bring my team on board with my plan, because – as you can imagine – this wasn't the first headache I'd ever given them. 'Here's Simon wanting to do something

---

[19] '"Designer" baby to save boy with blood disorder', *The Mail on Sunday*, 15 July 2001.

impossible, *again*. We'll have to create a load of new protocols, consent forms, patient information documents, and so on – all so he can chase after a dream.' But they saw what a big deal this was and – miracle on miracles – I managed to gain approval from the regulator too.

I was aware, though, that a serious ethical consideration was at stake and that once we'd announced our plans we'd have to brace ourselves for a backlash. I wasn't surprised when a slew of media articles appeared condemning us for what we were doing, with some commentators accusing us and the Hashmis of creating a baby for 'spare parts'. These included Robert Winston, who said the newborn baby 'would be beholden to the older sibling and could not be a child in its own right.'[20] However, I was confident the Hashmis would love any saviour sibling with all their heart, and in any case already wanted another child. I could also see it wasn't right to deny Zain the chance of a full and healthy life. The 'spare parts' analogy was incorrect because the stem cells would be taken not from the baby but from the foetal cord tissue that would be thrown away after the birth. Nor were we aiming to produce a 'designer baby', because we weren't intending to manipulate the embryo in any way.

So we treated Shahana and created some embryos, but didn't find a match. We were about to treat her again but the pro-life group CORE took out an injunction against us and the HFEA which forced us to put it on hold. To do this to a woman in her late thirties was effectively handing a potential death sentence to her sick son. Eventually the case went all the way to the House of Lords, which agreed the treatment was appropriate. Victory – but too late for Shahana. We tried stimulating her ovaries again but she couldn't produce enough eggs. Cruelly, her window of opportunity had closed.

---

[20] 'Making babies', *The Sunday Times*, 7 October 2001.

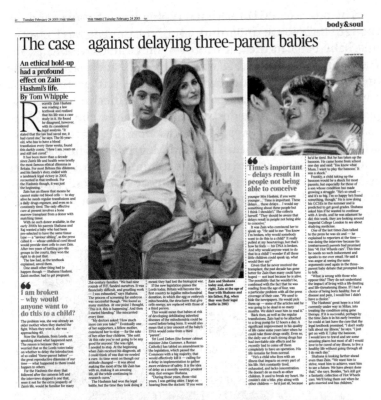

Figure 7.1: The case against delaying three-parent babies, *The Times*, 24 February 2005

This was the UK's first saviour sibling attempt. It failed but at least the HFEA and the House of Lords had established we were right to try. Shahana and her husband were pioneers and enabled us to establish our saviour sibling IVF programme in the UK. In fact, some time later there was the first NHS funded treatment for PGD and HLA tissue typing (the technical term), resulting in a national policy that funds up to three cycles for couples with genetic conditions (although there is still no national policy just for IVF). I've never been able to find out how much it costs to look after a child with beta thalassaemia, for instance, but it doesn't take a genius to realise it's considerably more than IVF and embryo screening combined, and I'm sure that's partly why this happened. A saviour sibling is doing two things: helping its parents have a healthy child, and helping them to cure the child who has the disease and who will always be a cost to the NHS.

The story of PGD for tissue typing has a happier ending, though. In 2010 we undertook another case that was to be the first baby born in the UK through the same technique as the Hashmis had wanted. He was called Max and was to be the brother of a little girl called Megan. She was profoundly ill and had been out of school a long time; her prognosis was poor. Her parents were desperate for a 'saviour sibling' for her so we created an embryo which was a perfect match and free of the genetic disease that affected Megan. After he was born, a stem cell transfusion from Max's umbilical cord took place and Megan regained her health, went back to school, and lived a normal life. She even sailed around the UK for charity as a teenager.

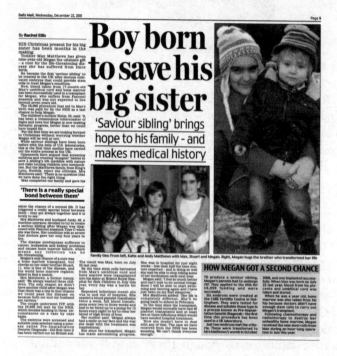

Figure 7.2: 'Boy born to save his big sister', *Daily Mail*,
22 December 2010

Her parents told me that when Max was a young boy he said to his sister, 'You know those stem cells I gave you? I think I should have them back now.'

'But don't you remember, Max?' retorted Megan. 'I gave you My Little Pony instead.'

Luckily Max agreed this was a fair exchange.

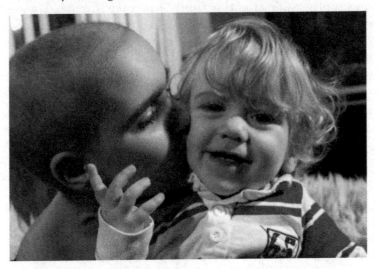

Figure 7.3: Megan kisses Max

It's never kids who have the problem, is it? It's only us who burden them with our judgementalism. The case of Megan and Max was one of those wonderful ones where I could get on with helping people through using technology that both worked and was allowed. If only they were all like that.

***

Not long after the controversy and heartbreak of the Hashmis' case, I was on a train to London. Occupied with typing a report into my laptop with all the frenzied concentration I could muster in a packed carriage, my phone rang. I was tempted to leave it but I was glad didn't when I heard what the man at the other end had to say. He was a lovely Scottish fellow called Alan Masterton and told me the tragic story of what he and his wife Louise had been through. They had four sons and had tried for years to have a girl because they thought she would be a wonderful addition to their family. They were eventually blessed with the birth of Nicole. For the first three years all was well, but one sunny day the children were playing in the garden with a helium balloon. The boys accidentally let it go near a bonfire and it burst into flames, burning Nicole terribly. She was rushed to hospital, but after two months she died. As Alan told me this his voice started breaking with tears, and thoughts of my own four children came to mind. I could only contemplate the unimaginable grief this family was going through. He went on to describe how he and Louise had tried to live with their guilt and also their anger towards the boys, even though they knew it wasn't the boys' fault. The boys themselves were eaten up with sorrow and regret, and the collective guilt was on the verge of destroying their beautiful family. They'd had medical and psychiatric help, but it could only go so far.

Eventually, Alan told me, he and Louise came to the conclusion that to have another daughter would create some kind of healing in their family. They knew this could never replace Nicole but that it would help them to move forward with their lives. This was supported wholeheartedly by their psychiatrist and their GP. There was a problem, though: Louise had been sterilised after the birth of Nicole, and even if she hadn't been, there was no way of them guaranteeing she would have a girl. 'Could you do this for us – help us have a girl?' he pleaded. I closed my laptop and thought for a moment, but soon realised there was no choice for me to make – it was yes.

'Leave it with me, Alan. I'll see what I can do but I can't guarantee anything. The HFEA will have to approve it because sex selection in embryos isn't allowed unless for serious health reasons. I see your case as a health reason because it's your mental health at stake and medical opinion is on your side, but not everyone will agree with me.'

My first step in a situation like this would normally have been to take the case to our external ethics committee, but I knew there was no point doing that until the HFEA had given it a general seal of approval first. So I went straight to the regulator with my argument. Its view was that it was the responsibility of the ethics committee to endorse it before it would consider the case, but that if the committee agreed my argument would probably succeed on medical grounds; in other words, it passed the buck but gave me hope. When I brought it to the ethics committee it was divided on the issue but eventually agreed I could go ahead because of the conclusive medical reports. Buoyed by this, I returned to the HFEA with the good news.

It said no.

Why allow me to raise the Mastertons' hopes and delay things by months, if it was going to block me all along? It was obvious the regulator was assuming, or hoping, the ethics committee wouldn't pass the case so it wouldn't have to make a decision. By now Louise was a year older, with every passing month making it less likely we'd succeed with IVF. There was no point brooding on it, though. Swallowing my anger and frustration, I worked out what to do next. The couple could still try for a baby, which would need to be by IVF because Louise had been sterilised, but they couldn't select the gender in the UK. I gained agreement from a clinic in Italy that I'd worked with before that – given our ethics committee was in support of me – it would determine the sex of the embryos for the couple. So the Mastertons drove all the way to Rome, producing a male embryo which they donated to an infertile couple, and two female ones which were implanted. Sadly Louise didn't become pregnant, a situation made more likely because of her age, and they had to abandon any hopes of having a girl.[21]

In 2001, following a year-long investigation by the parliamentary ombudsman, the couple received an apology from the HFEA for mishandling their case although it didn't overturn its decision. Interestingly, in 2003 the regulator also announced the results of its public consultation on sex selection for non-medical purposes: approximately 80 per cent of the 600 respondents said it shouldn't be allowed. For the Mastertons, at least they got the opportunity to try, and let's not forget it was the view of professionals associated with the case that they had medical grounds for selection. In the end Alan changed his career and trained as a solicitor so he could challenge these kinds of regulatory decisions, and also appeared on a BBC Two documentary.[22] He still keeps in touch with me from time to time and has always spoken incredibly warmly about what we did for his family. I suppose I have to be content with knowing I did my best, even when it wasn't good enough.

***

The world of IVF, and medical science in general, can be an uneasy marriage of altruism and commerce; just like a couple who've been together for years, either side can be the lead partner at times. This is something I discovered early on when I was a post-graduate student at Cambridge, decades ago. There, commercial matters were never, ever spoken about, and the

---

21 'Couple abandon attempts to have IVF baby girl', *BioNews*, 24 January 2005, www.bionews.org.uk/page_89538
22 *Fertility Tourists*, BBC Two, 6 March 2001.

idea of making money out of a scientific development was a complete no-no. I became frustrated when academics would discover something new only to see it being exploited by industry and with no benefit coming back to the institution. For instance, Cambridge University was where monoclonal antibodies were first developed – a huge leap forward in the treatment of disease. This generated billions for pharmaceutical companies but the hapless researchers who made the discovery still had to apply for grant funding year after year in the hopes of keeping their jobs. I thought this was bloody awful and hatched a plan to tackle it by writing a letter to the Secretary of State for Health, Patrick Jenkin.

> It's time the government woke up to the fact that academics do brilliant things, but neither they nor their institutions benefit from the commercial value of them. It always comes down to who patents the discovery first, which usually is a pharmaceutical or some other commercial company. In the meanwhile, academics get nothing. I suggest an independent body be set up for academics when they carry out a new development. It would drive the value for that piece of work, and the money coming out of it would be divided between the academic institute, the commercial organisations making use of it, and the academics themselves. This would create an additional incentive for researchers to develop new treatments, and valuable discoveries for humanity.

A couple of weeks after I'd posted off the letter with a flourish I was summoned to the office of Chris Polge, the head of my unit. He wore the expression of a man who was trying to look serious while suppressing a smile. 'Simon, we have a problem', he said. 'Did you write to the Secretary of State for Health?' I was proud to announce I had. 'Well, I've just had my knuckles rapped by the government. Can I suggest, next time you come up with a bold idea you refrain from using our headed notepaper to write it on? Even better, keep it to yourself.'

I'd been told. But ironically a year later Harvard University announced it was starting to do exactly what I'd proposed and eventually became a world leader in generating commercial income.

You may wonder what this has to do with CARE twenty years later. At that time I was contacted by OvaScience, a company created on the back of many years of research by scientist Jonathan Tilly. He profoundly believed, and had the data to prove, that women's ovaries contained not just a set number of eggs that are used up by the time the menopause arrives, but also stem cells that are capable of producing more. This was a ground-breaking discovery, because if those stem cells could be triggered to produce more eggs, women could have fresh eggs no matter what age they were. Imagine the potential for prolonging female fertility this represented. I wasn't the only person who was impressed. When OvaScience became a public company, its stock market offering quickly surged with a book value per share of 20.13 dollars in 2012, and they raised in excess of 200 million dollars.

Scientific observation states one of the reasons womens eggs decline as they get older is down to the mitochondria (the energy source in the cells) dying off. OvaScience, believing in Tilly's observations which were still highly conjectural, announced it was the only one able to find stem cells in the ovaries of an older woman with poor quality eggs, extract the young, fresh mitochondria from the stem cells, and transfer the stem cell mitochondria into the eggs of that same woman while she was undergoing an IVF procedure. It would be like putting new batteries into her ageing eggs. That woman could then have babies just as if she was younger – amazing. OvaScience asked me to test it further, which I thought was a great idea as it would allay my inner doubts, especially as I insisted the company fund the trial and ask the HFEA for approval. In theory I didn't need the regulator to give permission for my research as it doesn't adjudicate on the use of mitochondria on their own, only the whole egg when it's being fertilised. But without its endorsement I wouldn't be able to put the mitochondria into another egg and transfer it back into the woman, which was the whole point of the treatment. Once we went public about the trial, a flurry of email enquiries landed in my inbox from women desperate to take part, and soon I had more than 200 hopeful cases waiting. I told them they'd have to stay on hold until the regulator agreed we could go ahead, but that I hoped this would be before too long.

In the meanwhile, despite scientific protests to the contrary, the company began to carry out cases in Dubai, Canada, and Japan. The treatment wasn't cheap at 20,000 US dollars a cycle on top of the charge for IVF. A year went by and I still hadn't heard anything from OvaScience about the HFEA approval, and I was worried about the potential patients who kept wanting to know what was going on. They, and their eggs, were getting older so I asked what had happened with the application for a licence. I was told it was in progress and to keep the patients on standby. Eventually, after getting no further with OvaScience after several months more, I called the head regulator at the HFEA myself. He sounded puzzled. 'What application are you talking about?' he said.

'The OvaScience one, of course.'

'There isn't an application from them. OvaScience pulled it long ago.'

Astonished, I asked OvaScience what was going on. 'It's merely a temporary technical hitch – don't worry.' But when I looked into the company and discovered its board members had all changed recently, the penny dropped. There had obviously been a shift in strategic direction at the top and I concluded the business was scared the HFEA would turn down the company's application. Far better for the share price for the business to hold a technology with potential, than to have one that's been blocked by regulation. This made me furious, especially when I had to email each of the women who'd been waiting to explain I couldn't help them after all. I could only imagine their despair when they read it.

So I never managed to trial this exciting, and as yet unproven, development in the UK although it's available in some parts of the world. If I'd been able to undertake it and put the research into clinical use it would have shown the power of fundraising for a valuable new treatment. But it also demonstrates the dark side of commerce and the flip side of financially incentivising research while also operating in a regulated environment. The tragedy is, we can't now try it formally and therefore can't know for sure if it works because OvaScience's research data is shrouded in commercial secrecy. Also the financial markets have caught on, as the company, having raised and spent 200 million US dollars, has a value per share languishing at 1.4 dollars.

Although the trial of the OvaScience process didn't work out for us I've always been a huge fan of new technology in general. A few years ago, our Director of Embryology at CARE, Alison Campbell, became aware of a new innovation: time-lapse imaging machines. These film embryos while they remain sealed and protected in the high-tech incubator, thereby replacing the manual process of taking them out once a day to see if they're ready for putting back into their mothers. Not only does this mean we can inspect them without disturbing them, we can also see what they are doing while hidden from human sight. Alison was impressed and keen for us to buy one, but at 100,000 US dollars an incubator it wasn't an easy decision. I could, however, see the potential for it to change our understanding about early dividing embryos as well as improve the way we cared for them. If Alison would commit to tracking the data about embryo development provided there was a clear research element, we could go ahead. She agreed, and in 2011 we became the first UK clinic to install one. Later we also became the first to publish scientific papers questioning whether particular development patterns of embryos were related to normal or abnormal chromosomes; this was exciting to us because the cameras gave us a non-invasive way of examining the embryos.[23]

***

A cell is the most fascinating thing you can imagine; it's the single, contained unit of life. Not long ago I met up with a colleague in London, Mark Hughes, one of the pioneers of PGD technology. As we strolled down the hectic street, with people zig zagging around the traffic and car horns blaring, I said:

> Mark, just stop a minute. Look around us. Look at the activity. The people, the cars, the commuters, the energy created here. It's nothing – nothing – compared to what goes on inside a single cell. Proteins being made, carbohydrates growing, amino acid chains forming – they're constantly being built up and broken down, and signalling to other cells. Membranes communicating with cytoplasms, the formation and dissolution of a nucleus, the DNA being changed and dividing as it does so. It's unbelievable.

And that's just a single cell – we slough off thousands of them every time we brush our teeth and replace two million per second. We have fifty trillion in our bodies, each of them

[23] Campbell, Fishel et al 2013a, 2013b, 2014; Fishel, Campbell et al 2017, 2018.

busying themselves with countless activities all the time. And when we look at embryos using our time-lapse camera we can see their cells going through the most amazing changes.

Did you know that if I was to take a four-cell embryo and separate out each of those cells, it would turn into four embryos? This tells us each cell, at this early stage two days after fertilisation, has its own programme. Each one can make a baby. At the eight-cell stage, twenty-four hours later, we can't do that because the cells are starting to become different. They're losing the potential to become 'everything' and are growing to be mutually dependent on one another. By early on the fifth day, what do we have? About thirty to sixty cells, but they're made up of a few cells in a tiny ball in the middle with the rest on the outside, and a tiny cavity of fluid forming. That's a blastocyst. Those few balls of cells in the middle may – if we're lucky – make a baby, and the cells on the outside will form the placenta. It's unbelievably beautiful.

We know these cells are developing rapidly, the fluid volume is increasing, and, when we watch the embryo, we see it collapsing and expanding. What on earth can one single inspection of an incubating embryo, lasting a few seconds, tell us about what it will do an hour later or did an hour earlier? Nothing. But now we've got this time-lapse technology we've learned things we never knew before. For instance, we might view an embryo and see it's got to the stage of development we'd have expected at that point. But what we'd never have realised without the cameras is that, upstream, it had split into two cells, fused back into a single cell, and then exploded into four. This is called reverse cleavage and is abnormal so we wouldn't implant that embryo. Statisticians say our work demonstrates that time-lapse provides an independent, objective approach that's far superior to visual assessment alone. These cameras, if used properly, are revolutionising the way we do IVF.

Because only 35 per cent of embryos end up making a baby, we're constantly looking for ways to identify and select those which are in that group. After several years of studying the millions of images of embryo development, we can now be far more accurate when deciding which of a batch stands the best chance of success. We've come up with an algorithm that essentially goes like this: if an embryo has done x by x time more often than not it will create a baby. And if it's done y by x time it probably won't. The value of algorithms is they're independent of embryologists' personal opinions and preferences. Our first scientific paper of a trilogy on proving the value of this technology was in October 2017, and showed a 20 per cent increase in our live birth rate when using this algorithm. In October 2018 we published our second which showed that not only did we achieve better results with time-lapse over standard incubation, but that we could rank the embryos into four categories. Our third paper describes how much this objective approach outperforms the four decades-old way of assessing embryos subjectively.

We called this technology CAREmaps, and have now spent a million pounds replacing our standard incubators with time-lapse ones. Although we have the same 'box' as other places, we use ours far more extensively than most, which was my aim right from the beginning. I didn't want it to just be a fancy camera that took pictures, I wanted it to really work for us. Now we've been working with CAREmaps for seven years, recording more than 3,000 babies and observing millions of images, we've produced the world's first time-lapse human embryology atlas. As a bonus, we can give couples a recording of their embryo cells dividing while in the incubator, enabling them to start a photo album from the moment their egg was fertilised.

I smile when I compare my Bourn Hall days to now. There I spent hours each week visually inspecting embryos lying at an angle in a test tube placed in a glass jar, which was pumped with an air mix and placed in a warm cabinet. Now I put a dish into an incubator and don't even touch it for five days. We can even watch the embryos growing on our tablets or smartphones, or on a big screen in the lab.

One of the other major changes since Bourn Hall has been the increased consistency in embryology practice. Then, if I thought an embryo looked viable it would be implanted. But who's to say I was basing it on the right principles time after time? Doctors and scientists can interpret one set of patient notes in multiple different ways. This is why the algorithmic approach that CAREmaps allows is so helpful, because it removes some of the decision-making from researchers and medics. It's also why artificial intelligence should be used more, and why I'm working on incorporating it into my work as much as I can. In the next few months I expect to change a large portion of the way conventional embryology is carried out at CARE so that it's more consistent and objective. Of course a doctor's clinical experience has value, but informative data is more useful. If I can eventually move to a system in which the best protocol for a patient is decided by a click on a computer running an algorithm, I'll have achieved my aim.

Even though we have more data now to help us, the whole of IVF is still blighted by inconsistencies, not only in how embryos are graded but also in how they're implanted. This is why the next welcome development will be robotics. It sounds terrible to say, but a patient is lucky if she has a good obstetrician and unlucky if she doesn't. A robot, however, never has a bad day. Nor does it sneeze or need to pee at an inopportune time or have to pick up the phone to his or her spouse between cases because there's an urgent problem at home. Robotics only requires economies of scale to happen.

***

As I mentioned before, when I first started CARE I just wanted to make it viable. I never intended for it to become bigger than just one clinic and certainly didn't understand things like budgets and commercial operations too well, having been protected from that at the university. However, I suppose I should have known better than to assume it would ever be a one-site operation because it's not in my nature to turn an opportunity down. This came to pass a year after we opened, when I realised we were receiving a quarter of our patients from the north-west of the UK. When I looked into the reason why, I discovered there were only one or two units in that region, and with poor results. To rectify this, in the summer of 1999 we established CARE Manchester in an annexe to the Alexandra Hospital.

Then we looked further afield and realised many other practitioners were not practising IVF so well or wanted to expand their opportunities, and started discussions with a clinic in Northampton which we bought out. The following year I met Professor Ian Cooke, Head of Obstetrics and Gynaecology at Sheffield University and his scientist colleague Dr Liz Lenton, who'd been awarded a grant to investigate women's natural cycles. He'd purchased a terraced house in Sheffield with the money and opened up an IVF clinic for the joint purpose of research on this and treatments. About to retire in 2001, he was keen to sell, so we ended up acquiring that too. Our four clinics in Nottingham, Manchester, Northampton, and Sheffield became the core of what we re-named the CARE Fertility Group which has now produced 30,000 babies.

What drove me then, and continues to motivate me now, was and is to keep bringing in new developments if I think they will help our patients. If they can open up an opportunity for those who have nothing left to try, then all the better. We never want to say to anyone, 'Sorry, we don't have the technology or expertise to treat you for that.' That means CARE has to be cutting edge: if something can be offered we'll find a way to make it available. And once we've pioneered a new treatment we publish our findings so everyone in the field can benefit.

Of course expansion brings with it the challenge of making sure everyone follows a standard set of protocols, no matter where they're based. When we reached four clinics, here's what I and my team came up with to guide us:

- We will always offer best practice but we won't be dictatorial or dogmatic about it; if other clinics have better way of doing things than us, we'll learn from them.
- We will do our utmost to offer our patients everything available in the field, with stringently trained staff.
- We will never hide from our mistakes; they will happen, especially when we're being inventive, but we will be open about them whatever the cost because trust is everything.
- Our patient experience will be par excellence.

Given we've expanded mainly by taking over existing clinics, you can imagine how difficult it's been to bring people who've been working in their own way for years into line with our ethos. In the early days I found myself taking the softly-softly approach, wanting to coax people around in their own time. After two decades of further expansion, though, I've discovered this never works. To create a multi-site, best-practice operation working under an overarching brand has required tough measures at times. I think this has been my main challenge of recent years, and although it's been frustrating it's also been a fantastic learning curve.

I'm clear on one thing: you can either be ordinary, staying where you are and maybe slipping backwards in comparison with others, or you can be different. I don't believe Ken, Simon, and I have created such a successful group of clinics by chance. In 2012, CARE became the largest IVF group in the UK and was also the first to be sold to private equity investors that same year. In the beginning we were just a group of medical scientists who knew a bit about building IVF clinics; now we've created a professional enterprise, with the extra funding enabling us to expand into nine full clinics with another nine satellites. Expansion has given us economies of scale, which means we can invest in cutting-edge equipment and examine data from more patients. With 5,000 clients providing research material each year, we can do real research. And being big means we're more easily recognised by the pharmaceutical companies, medical research businesses, universities, and technology companies – they want to work with us because they know our size means we can deliver results quickly. This has led to all our clinics being in the top ten of the HFEA's measurement of success table with two of them at the number one and two spots. In a roundabout way I've achieved what I envisioned with Nurture, and what I originally wanted to do with Bourn Hall.

In 2017 I received an email from Ernst and Young telling me I'd been nominated for their Entrepreneur of the Year award. I assumed it was either a joke, a mistake, or one of those spam emails. Knowing our private equity partner, Bowmark Capital, was familiar with this kind of thing, I asked it whether I should take the nomination seriously. The answer was a definite yes. To be honest I found it a bit embarrassing – I'd never thought of myself as an entrepreneur before, let alone one who'd win an award. Imagine my surprise when I was voted the regional winner. I suppose it was because my entrepreneurship in the IVF world has always been fuelled by me pushing the boundaries of what's possible.

I know what will happen next. Worldwide IVF practice will end up being funded by some form of private equity, and eventually global funds will wade in. For instance, I'm currently advising various funds that are buying up small clinics across Europe with the aim of creating a big group with an overarching brand. When they're big enough, an even larger player will swallow them up into a more substantial pan-European or global brand.

What does this mean for patients? Nearly fifty years ago it took almost a decade to achieve a successful pregnancy from crude IVF technology. As time has moved on we've gone from laparoscopy to ultrasound-guided egg collection; from a ten-day hospital stay to a visit of a couple of hours; from infertile men only having the option of donor sperm to now conceiving their own genetic child; and from parents knowing nothing about their embryo's genetics to the introduction of screening and testing. Each of these has been introduced more quickly than the one before, with more and more babies and families as a result – the chance of having a baby through IVF has trebled since the early 1980s. And yet almost all of it has been made possible by the commercial world, either at private clinics or by patients funding their own treatment, or both. Given the most fearsome enemy of those struggling to conceive is time, it's not commercial pressure that creates the obstacles to progress but the slow, mundane nature of much clinical practice.

IVF is a business, but that side of it has never been my driver. My only purpose has been to improve people's lives through giving them the children they yearn for, and to do this I've ensured we can do amazing things by being both commercially successful and properly governed. It works both ways: the more patients I can treat, and the more innovative and cutting-edge technologies I can provide, the bigger the company grows. As long as we do this in a well-managed and ethical way, the more quickly both we and our patients can achieve their goals.

Chapter 8

The DNA of IVF

When Bob Edwards and Patrick Steptoe were travelling on their ten-year journey to develop IVF, they never doubted the ethics of what they were doing. If they could create a technology that would help people, it just made sense to try. And thank goodness they did, because the technique they spawned has inspired the creation of eight million babies around the world.

However, ethical controversies are intrinsically bound up with IVF – you could say they're in its DNA. Even before Louise Brown was born in 1978, Bob and Patrick found themselves defending their work from prominent people who denounced it as evil or misguided: doctors, scientists, religious leaders, politicians, and social commentators of every hue. It was predicted to be the thin end of the wedge, leading all the way to Armageddon. Children would suffer terrible psychological problems or birth defects which would be the fault of monster scientists 'playing God'. As the technology has allowed us to do more and more, so the voices of opposition have risen. Some of the questions they've asked have been interesting: when, if ever, is it allowable to select an embryo based on its sex or health? Are there certain people who shouldn't be given IVF? And where do we draw the line when it comes to manipulating embryos' genetic make-up? These are valid points, but whenever the cry of 'It's a step too far!' goes out I have to ask, 'A step too far for whom?' For the couple without a baby? For the mother and father who are watching their child die of a debilitating disease? Maybe, just maybe, it's for the parents to make that decision, not for anyone else.

As always happens, what was once novel and shocking has now become the norm, and nowadays IVF is almost entirely accepted except from within strict religious quarters. I'm still waiting to see where the harm of it is. Of course not all children grow up in happy families, but that will happen both with and without IVF. To me, nobody has the right to tell someone else how to live their life or decide what's right for them except in the rarest of circumstances. The way a person reproduces is not the business of anyone but them, and especially not of the government. As long as that person's intentions are well thought-through and medically sound, I can't see what's wrong with it. Even if I could, who am I to judge? I've seen so many childless couples suffer simply because society's rules have restricted their access to treatment, and who's to say which party is right or wrong – the couple or society? When I tried to give the Hashmis a baby so their son Zain could be treated for beta thalassaemia, for instance, I couldn't predict the long-term outcome for that newborn but I could know how hard we debated what it might be like for them. I took the common-sense view their parents would love them so much they wouldn't ever allow them to feel as if they were a bundle of 'spare parts'.

Sometimes I think the regulator only feels comfortable when it has objections to work with. When it allowed a saviour sibling for the Megan and Max case, for instance, this was on the basis that the embryo itself had a valid reason for being screened because it might carry the disease in question. But there exist diseases such as leukaemia, for which stem cell transfusion from a donor can provide a cure, but which can't be screened for in an embryo. When we became known as a clinic that could tissue match embryos, couples came to us who had children with conditions like leukaemia and for whom a match couldn't be found. In the HFEA's wisdom, it restricted the saviour sibling cases we were allowed to carry out to those in which the embryo itself had a disease we could test for. That meant we had to turn away patients asking for technology to help their sick child.

Another example is when a disease isn't guaranteed to cause problems in later life (so-called 'non 100 per cent penetrance'). I debated this with John Humphrys on the *Today* programme on

BBC Radio 4, talking about a family in which a young mother, whose own mother and both aunts had died of breast cancer, had understandably had both her breasts removed to make sure she stayed cancer free. Doctors were allowed to carry out that surgery but were not allowed to test her and her husband's embryos for that very same condition, because there was only an 80 per cent chance that if their baby had the relevant gene it would develop cancer. You read that correctly: 'only' 80 per cent.

This angers me because it forces parents to keep rolling the reproductive dice in an attempt to create a match sibling, and in the process possibly give birth to more babies with the same disease. Month after month, year after year they try, watching their child become sicker and sicker and eventually die. And for what? So people can say, 'At least we didn't allow the thin end of the wedge.' Given there are about 20,000 human genetic disorders, of which most can now be detected and screened in embryos, this is an issue we need to face up to.

It's not as if in any of these cases we proceed in a gung-ho way. Before going ahead we have independent counselling and a detailed consulting process for referring patients to specialists. I also wouldn't want to give the impression I have no limits; I've turned away couples when I felt it wasn't safe to give them IVF for either physical or mental reasons. And I've always relied on my external ethics committees, whatever clinic I've been running. These valuable bodies have grappled with all sorts of thorny issues, such as when a man wanted donor eggs and a surrogate to bear his child. Given we treat single women with donor eggs, the committee thought, why not a man? And given he can't physically carry the child, why not a surrogate? Should he be discriminated against because he's a man, not a woman? Given there have been plenty of cases over the years in which a woman has had a surrogate, sometimes from within her own family, the panel didn't feel it made sense to refuse the man's requests. Although we naturally have to take into account the best welfare of children born through interventive technology, we must do so without being unduly prescriptive.

In all of this I can never forget my pioneer patients, without whom no advances could have been made. Back in the 1980s I was helping out some colleagues in Johannesburg, South Africa, when they carried out the world's first implantation of an embryo into its grandmother (her daughter wasn't able to carry the baby herself). The press was camped outside the hospital, much like it was outside the one in Oldham when Louise Brown was born, and every detail of the patient's treatment became public property. For the courage of her, and people like the Hashmis, the Mastertons and many others, I have nothing but admiration.

Why do infertile couples go through this? What gives them the strength? Because, they tell me, without children they feel 'genetically dead'. Being able to pass on our genes is an instinct that runs deeply through our human psyche and I've even known some people to commit suicide if they can't have a baby. I remember when my father died, my sister and I saw him in his coffin. As Ruth kissed him during his final breaths, she murmured, 'Bye-bye Dad. You live on in Simon and me.' This was a huge comfort to us all, but for couples who can't have their own children this consolation is missing – the end of their lives is the end of their line.

When IVF doesn't work it's desperate of course, but it means a huge amount to the couples to have tried and failed than never to have tried at all. It helps them to gain some closure. This poses a problem for me because if a patient has virtually no chance of success I ask myself if I should do the treatment anyway. If I say no many will take this as a cue to try elsewhere, possibly in a country where there are fewer ethical considerations and more chances of being exploited. I've had letters from patients who've had 'treatment' in the Middle East, for instance, and have paid unbelievably large sums before they learn they can't be helped after all. This is abusive and seeing the tactics of these bad practitioners was one of the reasons I set up the IVF degree course at Nottingham University. I also had a flash of inspiration in 1997 when I set up an 'ask the doctor' email address for couples to ask anything they wanted about IVF. I offered free advice to anyone from anywhere, and the questions I was asked helped me understand just how far the problems go. Because IVF fails more times than it succeeds it's easy for bad clinics to hide behind statistics when they explain their lack of success, but the reality is many countries don't regulate clinics and patients are exploited as a result. The email address is still up and running: it's simon. fishel@carefertility.com. If you want to ask me a question please feel free. Although I try to I can't promise to answer each one myself, but if you don't hear back from me, it will be from one of my medical directors.

People have taken a long time to come to terms with the technological changes in IVF and probably always will. Some will never accept them. Switzerland, for example, has only just changed the law to allow embryo screening for genetic diseases, and it's still illegal there to donate sperm directly. Over the years I've seen how our personal standards are largely dictated by our religious and social backgrounds; they're never truly our own. Some time ago I had the good fortune to share a speaking platform with Richard Dawkins, author of The God Delusion. We had a fascinating chat afterwards. His view is no child is born a Muslim, a Christian, or indeed any other religion, but is trained and conditioned to think along these lines as they grow up. I absolutely agree with that and always have. In fact, when my mother asked me if I'd ever give a Jewish patient an egg from a non-Jewish woman, I replied, 'Show me the Jewish gene.'

Right from the beginning, whenever I looked down a microscope at a sperm and an egg and the embryo they made, I could see no colour, race, or genetically-based prejudice. I saw only the hope of the parents of those cells. The couple's dream, and mine, was that the embryo would keep dividing and one day become their baby, entering the world they had waiting for it. This is why I try to put aside my own conditioned thinking when dealing with others, which has led me to have some strange thoughts at times.

One particular weekend at Bourn Hall there was a Palestinian chap and his wife being treated there along with an Orthodox Jewish couple. Both fathers were as anxious as anybody is throughout the IVF process, which helped them to bond while their wives were going through the endless process of having their urine tested every few hours. As I watched the men chatting away I mused on the imaginary outcome of a swapping of the men's sperm or even (and I held my breath here) the embryos. The couples were of the same broad ethnicity, so no-one would know. Of course I'd never, ever have done such a thing, but the mere thought of it brought home the artificiality of our ideas about culture and religion.

In the early days of CARE a highly successful Asian couple came to see me; the man was a professor of engineering, the woman a professor of mathematics. They needed an egg donation and asked if I could find an Asian donor. I said I thought I could, and when I'd managed to locate one I called them back in again. They arrived at my clinic beaming with excitement.

'Where does the donor come from?' the woman asked.

'Pakistan', I replied.

'Stop there. We can't possibly have a Pakistani donor –
        we're Brahmins. No Pakistani egg would be
        suitable for us.'

I was stunned. 'Hang on a minute', I said. 'We're talking genetics here. This child will look like your ethnic group, and in any case there's no such thing as a Pakistani or Brahmin gene.' The couple thought for a few moments. The husband responded, 'Could we use one of your ordinary donors? Because if we can't have a Brahmin donor, we'd rather have a Caucasian than a Pakinstani one.'

I was astounded. 'Okay, but this isn't my decision to take alone now. I'll have to bring it to my ethics committee, because what you're asking is to bring a child into the world who will stand out strongly in its community.' I knew from what the couple had already told me that they didn't mix much outside their Asian social group. 'This isn't just about you, it's about the welfare of the child.'

I took the case to the ethics committee and we agreed any request for trans-racial donation would always go to it first, with full pre-counselling for the couple. We wanted to make sure they understood the social consequences of a child growing up in a different ethnic environment to its own. Although I have a libertarian approach to my patients' wishes there's an extra consideration too, and that's the welfare of the child. In the case of this particular couple we refused their request, although we've carried out trans-racial donations in other circumstances.

Being Jewish, I'm often approached by other Jews for advice on IVF and having been to night school in my youth to learn more about Judaism and the Rabbinic deliberations on the biblical text (I wasn't particularly religious, I just liked the debates), I'm aware of how many ways there are of interpreting Jewish edicts. There's a saying: 'If you have ten rabbis, you have ten opinions', and even today our Jewish patients often seek their rabbi's advice before they come to me. This is exemplified by my experience of meeting a lovely, and extremely Orthodox, couple from London a few years ago. I could see how desperate they were to have a baby but their problem revolved around the fact that the man had no sperm, which meant his only option was to use a donor. Normally this wouldn't have been an issue but he was a member of the Cohanim. According to a 5,000 year-old Judaic tradition this is the high-level, priestly category of Jewish men and their families (in fact it's where the surname Cohen comes from). In practice the only way you'd notice a difference between the Cohanim and other Jews is at a particular point in the Orthodox service, at which the Cohanim and their male family members have a special role for a few minutes. But to this Orthodox couple the distinction was vital.

The man had asked his rabbi whether donor sperm was acceptable and the rabbi went away to consider it. Eventually he gave his verdict. 'The child will not be a Cohanim because they haven't come from your loins', he said.

> You can use donor sperm but only under one of the following conditions. You can announce your child's status to your community so everyone knows why, when you're in the synagogue, he isn't performing the Cohanim rituals with you. Or you can leave your community – maybe go abroad – and simply don't behave as a Cohanim; that way there'll be no separation between you and your child. Either option is acceptable.

Talk about forcing a couple between a rock and a hard place. The man and his wife were deeply embedded in their community and were devastated at the thought of choosing between staying near their family and friends and being accepted at their synagogue. However, I knew only a boy could follow in his father's Cohanim tradition, which meant a girl wouldn't attract the kind of attention the man was worried about. 'Let's think outside the box', I said. 'What if we gave you a girl?' The couple were delighted with the idea and went back to the rabbi with this solution. He gave it his blessing.

But here's where the problems started. Given sex selection for anything other than medical reasons is against the law in the UK, I went straight to the regulator. I knew I'd have a battle on my hands to persuade it to accept my thinking, but I was convinced it was a mental health issue for this couple to have a girl, and therefore permissible. Sadly the reply was no, which I thought was heartless. Today this couple are still childless, even though we could have given them a girl and they could all have lived a wonderful life.

What would you have done, I wonder? It's one of those stories everyone will have an opinion on, but you and I have the luxury of it being no more than a fascinating debate. For that couple it was a tragedy.

Keeping an open mind about cultural and religious issues has saved me from endless headaches over my career in IVF, because I can almost always fall back on my conviction that the patient knows what's best for them and their potential family. While I was at Nurture I held a clinic in Saudi Arabia a few times, and on one of my visits I had a consultation with a Saudi general. My sessions over there were always strange because the woman would be covered up and couldn't be spoken to, so I'd have to talk directly to the husband. If I wanted to know when his wife's last period was, for instance, I'd ask him and he'd give me the answer. Unfortunately the general's wife was forty-eight, so I had to deliver the bad news she'd be unlikely to conceive even with my help. They went away and I assumed that was the end of it. When I next returned to Saudi I was surprised to see the man sitting in my office again. This time there were two women in black veils, one on either side of him.

'Doctor', he said. 'You said this wife', pointing to his right, 'won't be able to have my baby. But I've got another wife here', pointing to his left, 'who is only nineteen'.

'That's more promising.'

'There's a problem. She's my second wife, and my first wife comes first. My primary wife must be the first to bear my child. Can you use the eggs from my second wife to give a baby to my first one? After that I can have babies with my second wife naturally.'

To my mind this was a genius solution, because although egg donation isn't allowed under Muslim law, this would be a wife-to-wife transfer. I could see what a social disgrace it would be for both him and his first wife not to have his first baby and agreed to do as he asked. The IVF was successful, with his first wife giving birth to a baby using the second wife's egg. After that he went on to have more babies with his second wife. All was well.

***

The amazing thing about IVF is not only can it help individual couples to have children, but it also allows us to offer a fertility solution to an entire group of people who have already suffered enough: childhood cancer sufferers. While I was at Nurture I came across a scientific paper explaining how children with cancer were now more likely to survive to adulthood, but would be unable to have children because of the treatment they'd undergone years earlier. I thought about how sad it would be for these people to grow up knowing they were infertile. What would it be like when starting a new relationship, for instance? How would they cope, knowing they couldn't have children of their own? This is where Nurture comes in, I thought. We'd already teamed up with various other medical and non-medical disciplines by then, so why not oncology too?

I gathered together a group of experts for a meeting at Nottingham University, at which I offered Nurture's facilities to store children's reproductive tissues for when they grew up. Although there was no way of using them then, I trusted that by the time these children reached adulthood we'd have cracked the problem of how to use them to restore fertility. For girls it was relatively simple because every girl is born with all her eggs which – at that time of her life – aren't capable of being fertilised. That meant I didn't need HFEA approval to extract and store them as the regulator only covers the use of viable eggs. For boys it was more tricky, although for a different reason. Before a boy hits puberty he doesn't manufacture sperm, so the only answer was to take some of his testicular tissue. Experiments with rats in the US had proved that immature tissue from the testes could produce sperm when transferred into the testes of an adult (sterile) hamster, which led me to believe the same would be possible for humans. It was exciting to think we could help these children but – frustratingly for me – it was shortly afterwards that I resigned from the university due to the funding issue with Nurture, and swiftly became persona non grata. Eventually it was left to researchers from Cambridge and Edinburgh to carry on my passion in this area.

In the meanwhile, in 1997, the potential to help these children was still playing on my mind when I received a phone call from a man called Ian von Memerty. He was a famous entertainer and producer in South Africa, and had been given my name by a South African TV company that had recently broadcast an interview with me. As he launched into his family history, I had to sit down to take it all in. When Ian and his wife Vivienne had first met, they weren't to know they were both carriers of a rare and abnormal gene that meant their children were at risk of inheriting a condition called mucopolysaccharidosis VI. This is a metabolic disorder causing tissues and organs to enlarge and become painfully inflamed, along with skeletal abnormalities. Sufferers don't tend to survive beyond their early twenties. After they married they had a daughter, Valeska, and noticed she was a little hard of hearing. Investigations for this led them to discover that, in a million to once chance, they both carried the gene that condemned her to an early and painful death. There was worse to come. By that time Vivienne was already pregnant with their second child, and they were given the dreadful news there was a one-in-four chance that the newborn would inherit the same condition. The possible saving grace was that if the new baby didn't have the disease it could provide the only potential cure for Valeska in the form of a bone marrow transplant – in other words, it could be a saviour sibling. Tragically this was not to be, because their son Oscar also turned out to have the disease. 'It was such a terrible time', said Ian. 'We went straight from finding out Valeska was ill to discovering Oscar had the same thing.'

This led Ian to search all over the world for a bone marrow transplant, as under South African law only a sibling could be a donor. Eventually he raised enough money to fly his family to Manchester in the UK for a year. Valeska's treatment seemed to work (although sadly she died two years later), so the couple's attention then turned to a transplant for Oscar. Their hopes revolved around him being able to live a full life including maybe having children one day, and the reason Ian called me was because he'd heard I was working on ways to preserve the fertility of children who'd be rendered sterile due to this kind of treatment. I replied that in theory I could help but in practice all the research for this so far had been on animals rather than humans, and that the UK regulator would have much to say about the matter. Strictly speaking I didn't need its permission as the procedure didn't involve the use of viable sperm, but I didn't want to take a chance. 'The HFEA tends to respond more quickly to members of the public, though', I told him. 'Why don't you contact it yourself?'

The next thing I knew I had a phone call from a journalist, Ian Munro. 'You know the von Memerty case? I suggest you look at The Times tomorrow.'

'Why?'

'Just buy it.'

The following day, 22 September 1997, on the front page of
The Times was the announcement that the HFEA had granted
permission for testicular tissue cells to be taken from boys
who needed chemotherapy that would otherwise render them
infertile. These cells would be frozen until they reached puberty
in the hope they could be used to 'repopulate' the testicles in
later life. I have to hand it to the HFEA; Ian had contacted them
on the Monday morning and by the Friday afternoon they'd
said yes. There was nothing to stop me going ahead.

Nothing, of course, apart from assembling a team of
specialists to carry out the procedure. This we proposed to do
while Oscar was having his bone marrow transplant in order
to avoid him going through repeat operations. Imagine being a
cancer surgeon due to operate on a seriously ill three-year old
boy, and along comes an IVF specialist asking if he can arrive in
your theatre to take a piece of the patient's seminiferous tubules
which would, when he was older, be the ones to manufacture
sperm. I'll be honest, there was a fair bit of hostility from
members of the cancer team, and I can't say I blame them. It
did seem far-fetched. They were also keen to establish how I'd
process the tissue once it was extracted because this required
extremely sterile conditions; the hospital had a sterile lab but
would they let me use it? My colleague Dr Irfan Aslam was
hugely helpful in persuading the hospital, and eventually we
got the green light from the surgeon, the operating theatre, the
hospital, and the lab.

Off we went to Manchester where, in the operating theatre,
the paediatric surgeon gave me the piece of Oscar's testicle.
Irfan and I prepared it in the lab as best we could, put it into the
deep freeze, and transported it to Nottingham. When Oscar was
confirmed as recovered from his condition it was the moment
to think about how the tissue could be used when he was old
enough and wanted a baby. One option was to put it into the
testes of a mouse because this had worked in animal tests; then
we could take it out again and use it to create an embryo through
sperm micro-injection. When this thinking went public it
generated a strange magazine cartoon portraying a human baby
wearing whiskers and a mouse outfit with a chunk of Swiss
cheese, with the caption 'Of mice and men'. The other option
was to transplant the tissue directly into Oscar's testes to see if
it would start working under his normal hormonal conditions.

The truth was, we didn't know what we'd do because it was far ahead of its time. As it stands, Oscar's testicular tissue is still sitting in our liquid nitrogen tanks at CARE, ready for when he wants it. Other scientists and doctors around the world have now started doing the same thing as the prospect of re-transplantation to the testis is becoming realistically close.

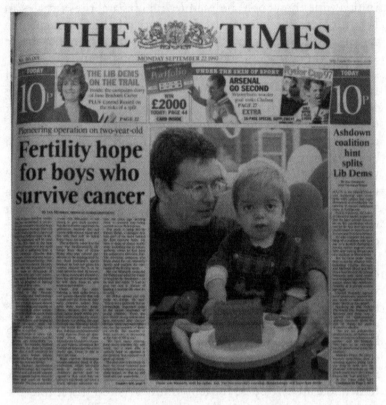

Figure 8.1: 'Fertility hope for boys who survive cancer', *The Times*, 12 September 1997

My experience with Oscar made me realise there was no funding available for this kind of research. I'd carried out the procedure for the von Memertys at no charge, but that wasn't sustainable and I knew, with infertility being so poorly funded generally, there would be little appetite from the government to support investigations for cancer patients. So I set up a foundation with the aim of researching the preservation of fertility in children made sterile through chemotherapy. I called it The Rachel Foundation, after Rachel in the Bible who was one of the first people on record to describe how it feels to be unable to have a baby. In Genesis Chapter 30, Verse 1, she casts up her heart-rending plea to God: 'Give me a child else I die!' I understood this cry as being more than just the desperation of someone who can't have children, it was also the grief of a woman who knows her family line will be no more. The pain of infertility is so devastating, it's not surprising the first recorded cry for medical help should be for that.

This was what was distressing an elderly man who I met when I was at Nurture. One of the nurses from the main hospital told me he'd been asking me to visit him at his sick bed, and although he was certainly not my normal kind of patient I said I'd go along. As I arrived at his bedside I saw a tired, wasted old man propped up on pillows. What would he have to say to me?

'Are you the doctor who does the fertility work?' he asked. 'I want to tell you my story.' He paused with a deep breath and didn't say anything for a moment or two. A guttural choke escaped from his mouth and I realised he was crying. After a while he composed himself enough to say, 'I've never been able to have children, and it's been the most terrible thing in my life. I don't have much but I do have a small house. With no family to leave it to, it's yours. Please take it for your research so you can help other people like me.' I was overwhelmed.

Sadly the bequest didn't come about as he passed away before he could make the arrangements, but it confirmed I'd done the right thing in setting up the Rachel Foundation. At least there would be somewhere people could donate to in future. It continues to this day, although it's never been well funded. I'm always touched when fundraisers run marathons or hold bake sales for it, and it's supported a number of research projects. It also means when a grateful patient wants to make a donation to an appropriate charity and asks which one, I can say The Rachel Foundation.

***

The ability to preserve a child's fertility, as we did with Oscar von Memerty, came about – like so many breakthroughs in IVF – by teaming up with experts from other disciplines and using their technology alongside ours. These discoveries aren't down to any individual genius, like the striker on the football field who scores the winning goal, but to a combination of specialists in different fields working as a team. When IVF takes a high-tech approach we do so as one in a chain of people who've pioneered the science that makes it possible.

A great hope for IVF has always been to acquire cells from early fertilised eggs, because only at this stage are embryos capable of creating all the other cells in the body. This is what's meant by 'stem cells'. If surgeons can use these early stem cells that are not yet imprinted with the code of any specific cell, they can be transplanted with no problem into a patient's body. It's now believed stem cells can be used to treat all sorts of degenerative organ diseases that simply require healthy cells to regenerate an organ, such as Parkinson's disease or many heart conditions. At one point I worked on a project with Sheffield University using embryos donated for research. From one single five-day embryo they were able to grow macular stem cells for the eye and store them. These cells have a theoretically indefinite life and are now being placed onto gossamer thin, non-reactive membranes behind the eyes of people going blind from macular degeneration. So those stem cells from one embryo are being used in clinical trials to restore the sight of countless people. Who could imagine IVF being party to curing blindness?

What's more, scientists are increasingly able to take other cells and 'de-programme' them so they become like stem cells. They can remove some of your skin cells, for instance, and take them back to their ancestral phase where they don't know they're 'you'. These skin cells can then be transformed into other tissues such as heart tissue. This means although stem cell technology is essential for the future of medicine, where the cells come from may not necessarily be embryos. Even more futuristically, but only around the corner, such cells may be transformed into egg or sperm cells – including from the opposing gender. So for men who can't produce sperm, we could take some of their other body cells, make sperm in a dish, and use that in IVF to give them children. Perhaps gay and lesbian couples could have a child without the intervention of a third-party gamete.

***

The future of IVF looks exciting and in the four decades since I started work at Bourn Hall live birth rates have tripled. In fact, for a young, healthy couple, natural conception is no longer a more efficient as a way of conceiving a baby than IVF. The chances of a highly fertile couple succeeding naturally in a single month is 25 per cent, and with IVF it's around 50 per cent. Of course, with IVF a patient can only try once every few months whereas there's nothing to stop a couple trying month after month in the natural way, so the comparison isn't absolute – but it's revealing. Because of this I'm often asked whether, due to the benefits of genetic screening in embryos, couples will opt for IVF as a default in future. I'm not sure if this will happen but I'm convinced most people wanting to conceive will at least opt for personal screening beforehand. Who knows, maybe this will progress to sex being kept for fun while technology is used for reproduction? Our descendants could have their genes screened at conception and at puberty their gametes stored, ready to whisk out of the freezer for when they want their own genetically screened baby.

This will be to the huge benefit of the human race or at least to those parts that can afford it. After all, we're now at the extraordinary point when we can wipe out certain genetic diseases from a family line. And we're on the cusp of one of the most heated debates ever: whether or not to edit the human genome to improve who we are. Could we call this evolution in action? And could we say to religious objectors this is 'doing God's work', in that it's improving the human condition? Is not modifying human DNA at the point of conception to correct the potential for a child to be born with Type 1 diabetes, for instance, simply twenty-first century medicine, just as heart transplants were the twentieth century's *cause célèbre*? Heaven knows what people in the Middle Ages would have thought of transferring the heart – the seat of our soul – from one individual to another. Think, also, of how we're already able to cure embryos of genetic diseases instead of just screening them; this means they're available to their parents rather than being discarded. Doing things that affect sperm, eggs, and embryos is different to operating on a whole person because it's what's known as germ line therapy; if it happens in the eggs and sperm it can be carried through to future generations. And that's precisely the point: a couple seeking a genetic remedy will no longer need to worry about their children or grandchildren having the same problem. Surely our efforts should be going towards ensuring the safety of the technology that can achieve this, rather than assuming that DNA is somehow sacred?

Part of this leap forward in genetic screening was the birth of the child in 2009 who would become known as Baby Oliver. IVF practitioners had known for years that early miscarriages are often due to an error in the embryo's chromosomes. The problem was the technology geneticists had until then only enabled them to look at nine pairs of chromosomes, and we have twenty-three. A company called BlueGnome, a spin-out from Cambridge University, developed a new approach to modern molecular genetics called bioinformatics. This is a mathematical study of genes and is changing the world of genetic technology. BlueGnome was looking at the main chromosomal abnormalities, such as those that cause Down, Edwards, and Patau Syndromes (chromosomes 21, 18, and 13 respectively), together with some others which are known to cause miscarriages. One of the scientists there, Tony Gordon, contacted me. He told me the company didn't have a way of analysing a single embryo cell, but that he could see the potential in it and would I be interested in working with them to develop this? Of course I would! I'd been searching for years for a better way of screening our embryos for chromosomal problems.

First Tony had to win over his reluctant colleague, Nick Haan, who was far from sure that IVF was something BlueGnome should be getting into. In fact he was pretty frosty about the idea. We went back and forth for ages, and in the end I said, 'Nick, if you give us this technology I'll give you a whole new world. Trust me.' Eventually he agreed. It took a year of us working with BlueGnome through 2008 before we were sure we were ready to go live, but we got to the point at which it was time to ask the HFEA to validate the BlueGnome laboratory as being licensed to carry out this work.

No sooner had my application gone in than a couple from London arrived in my clinic. They'd been through thirteen cycles of IVF, all of which had failed, including some due to miscarriages. The woman was in her early forties and with that history I'd normally have turned them away, but given we were about to trial this new technology I asked them if they'd be interested in being the first to give it a go. They had no hesitation in saying yes – it was their only hope. We extracted some eggs and screened the eggs genetically for the chromosome errors that would cause a miscarriage, and while we were waiting for the results, fertilised them and created some embryos. This is where it got interesting. She only had two good-looking embryos and a slow one that didn't look promising, but when the screening results came back the two good-looking ones turned out to be abnormal and the slow one okay. Normally I'd have implanted the 'good' ones, so this was a complete reversal of normal practice. To the couple's delight the chromosomally healthy embryo produced a baby, who they called Oliver.

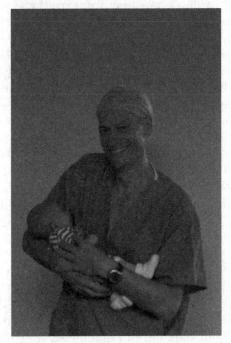

Figure 8.2: Baby Oliver

This was the first time the full twenty-three pairs of chromosomes in a human egg had been screened as part of IVF, and the story went viral all over the world. Array CGH Screening, as the technology is called, quickly became popular and moved into the screening of embryos as well as eggs. Only a few years later in 2012, BlueGnome was bought out by US company Ilumina for an 'undisclosed sum' estimated at over fifty million dollars mainly because of this new expertise. I'm still waiting for my drink from Nick!

But here's the research paradox again. After Baby Oliver was born there was much concern in the medical field that I hadn't carried out a randomised, controlled trial of the technology. This, said various experts, was the only way of proving whether it worked for sure. The way we'd done the test was to use what's called the 'polar body' of the egg. When a woman's eggs are formed each holds only half of the full set of forty-six chromosomes, because at fertilisation the sperm will provide the other twenty-three. However, when an egg cell divides upon fertilisation it has a dilemma. It needs to keep both sets of chromosomes (one from itself and one it gained from the sperm) and at the same time retain the nutrients and energy needed for those early cells to divide – this comes from the main body of the cell called the cytoplasm. The egg has therefore devised an ingenious way of having its cake and eating it: it shunts out the other half of the chromosomes into a tiny, pinched-off part of the cytoplasm called the polar body. Crafty! So when the sperm enters the egg there's a vast supply of nutrients and energy from which the newly fertilised egg can call to go through its next few rounds of cell division. We can make use of this tiny polar body by removing it, examining its chromosomes, and inferring the chromosomes that remain in the egg without touching the egg itself. It's like drawing on a mirror image of a person without touching the person themselves.

Following Baby Oliver we tried to publish an article on our first hundred cases, which was submitted to the *European Society of Human Reproduction*, or *ESHRE*. I was surprised, as was BlueGnome, when my abstract was rejected and discovered it was down to various people not liking the fact I'd raced ahead without the gold standard of randomised controlled trials. In other words, it was politics. *ESHRE* then announced it would do a controlled trial itself. And do you know what? Nearly ten years later it still hasn't published its results because it's run into the nightmare of funding and patient recruitment issues that bedevil all such experiments. What if I'd told Baby Oliver's parents we had a technology to help them but couldn't offer it until a randomised controlled trial had taken place? And that it may take ten years or even more than my lifetime? Imagine if Lesley Brown and her co-pioneering patients had been part of such a trial. Louise would not be here and I'd have no story to tell.

In fact, so fast does science speed ahead that a couple of years later we made a further breakthrough in preventing miscarriages. As far as we know there's one gene mutation in a man's DNA that causes a miscarriage in a woman; not only this, but it causes babies to be born small, gives high blood pressure to the mother in pregnancy, and induces complications with the placenta. Although several institutions around the world had been studying this gene, none had looked at how IVF could help solve the problem. CARE was the first to do that and my colleagues and I published three scientific papers on this, proving the gene is equally present in men and women attending our IVF clinics;[24] in fact, over 40 per cent of couples in that study carried it between them. If a woman comes to see us who's had multiple miscarriages, we test the blood of both her and her partner. That way we can give the right drugs to the woman to enable her to carry her baby to full term and remain healthy afterwards. With this treatment a woman has the same chance of having a baby as if she or her partner didn't have the defect, and without it she'd almost certainly miscarry or have a placenta-related problem. I'm currently working with some US scientists to develop the world's first test for screening embryos that may be carrying this gene, rather than just checking the parents' blood without knowing if the gene will be transmitted to the embryo. This will make it even more reliable.

It's now even possible to edit out some defective genes by making precise changes to living cells, through a technology called CRISPR-Cas9. Modifying genes, mutant or otherwise, isn't something that's yet allowed in humans but it can be done. As an aside, I've been asked by some prospective parents if I can edit out the teenage gene. I once did a news item for this for a local TV station as an April Fool's Day spoof, pretending new gene editing technology had finally allowed me to reach my professional goal of making parenthood of adolescents a smooth ride. I even had a name for it: the STROP gene. Wouldn't it be great if I could achieve it – the patent alone would be worth the work!

As you can see, IVF has moved way beyond simply giving babies to infertile people. It's now part of a web of technologies and processes that allow for the removal of unhealthy genes, the curing of older children with terminal illnesses, and the enabling of women to carry babies to full term. In the future it will also help women to delay the effects of the menopause

---

[24] Fishel, Rashmi et al. 2014; Fishel, Greer et al. 2016; Fishel, Baker et al. 2017.

and allow them to have babies later in life. We've all seen the increase in women using donor eggs, and around 50,000 a year do this in Europe alone. Some even freeze their eggs in case they want to use them later, a process which is by no means guaranteed to produce a pregnancy and involves multiple clinic visits along with lots of drugs. My ambition is to go several steps further than this by offering women the option of having part of their ovarian tissue removed instead. Ovaries are a bit like kidneys – women don't need two. Even so, if a strip is removed from one it doesn't do the work of the ovary any harm and the thousands of eggs contained in the removed strip can be frozen along with the ovarian tissue. This process can be done as a one-off procedure without the use of hormonal drugs – much easier than traditional egg collection. Of course the most obvious benefit is for women about to go through cancer treatment, who can freeze their tissue for when they've recovered. But other women can also use it as an 'insurance policy' so if they need the eggs when they're older they're there for them.

However, although the 'remove now and use later' element is a great benefit, it's not the main point of this procedure. If you are, or know anyone who is, going through the menopause you'll no doubt be aware of the miserable symptoms it can induce. There are also health risks built into this period such as cardiovascular disease and osteoporosis. By extracting a piece of ovarian tissue when a woman is younger and transplanting it back again later, we can put off the menopause by at least ten years. It provides a natural hormone replacement that's safer and more responsive than HRT, and prolongs the fertile period at the same time. You could say it kills two birds with one stone. And if there's a fuss about women having babies in their seventies as a result, the tissue can be implanted anywhere – in her armpit for instance – so it doesn't allow for pregnancy but still enables the menopause to be delayed.

I'm so excited by the potential of this that I've taken the plunge and gathered the best people together to form a company called ProFaM – Protecting Fertility and Menopause (and of course, all our work is pro-family). We have a professor from Birmingham University as our academic guru, a brilliant laparoscopic surgeon who has the skills to remove the tissue and transplant it back. I've also pulled in the world's foremost cryrobiologist in this area, Professor Christiani Amorim, who's been freezing reproductive tissues for nearly twenty years in

Belgium for cancer patients. ProFaM will be the first company in the world to freeze women's ovarian tissue for fertility preservation or menopause management, rather than because they're having cancer treatment. It could transform women's lives after fifty-five, and might eventually be seen as a national health and economic benefit; the medical expense in Canada for osteoporosis, for instance, is estimated to rise from 1.3 billion dollars in 1993 to 32.5 billion in 2018.

Chapter 9

The Legacy of IVF

It's amazing to think a technology that started out in a portacabin with a glass jar, a few petri dishes, and a box warmer, should have transformed into a high-tech industry that now contributes to solving major health problems around the world. I like to think the backbone of my work over the last forty years has been using the legacy of Bob Edwards and Patrick Steptoe in a way they could never have imagined. Now IVF isn't only about creating babies for infertile couples – a hugely rewarding aim in its own right – but also about improving the health of the human race.

On Bob's seventy-fifth birthday in 2000, I was invited to deliver a lecture at the Venice Lido covering some of his life, and finished it with a quote from Sigmund Freud.

> Humanity has in the course of time had to endure from the hands of science two great outrages upon its naive self-love. The first was when it realised that our earth was not the centre of the universe [...] The second was when biological research robbed man of his particular privilege of having been specially created, and relegated him to a descendant from the animal world. (Sigmund Freud, *Introduction à la psychanalyse*, 1917)

If Freud had been alive today I believe he'd have added a third 'outrage': that human procreation can no longer be considered solely the task of divine provenance. Not only can scientists manipulate the process of reproduction, but they can also monitor and forestall diseases for the overwhelming benefit of mankind. I know scientists are just people like everyone else, but I do like to think there was something divine in what Bob and Patrick initiated.

Most people think working in IVF means you wave goodbye to the results of your work when they're no bigger than a full stop. And sadly that's normally true, but some of my embryos have a habit of coming back into my life in the most marvellous ways. Laura Rush was one of these, and the seventy-fourth of the babies I created at the Park Hospital. She eventually returned to work there once it had become CARE Nottingham and was delighted to see a picture of herself as a four-cell embryo. She loved working in our clinic seeing how babies just like her were created and was inspired to become a chemist.

These blasts from the past also found their way into my family. In my early days at the Park Hospital we implanted two embryos – a boy and a girl – who later went on to become black belts in martial arts. The girl won seven international championships and still teaches today. I've always enjoyed martial arts and when one of my sons was young we wanted to do it together, but found it hard to find a club that would take both parents and children. I approached the girl's father and asked if she would open a club in my village. She did, and twenty years later it's still going strong. For years she was my teacher, although given the hell she put my body through there were times when I wished I'd not taken that petri dish out of the incubator!

One of the most transformative aspects of IVF is the way it's re-defined family life. At CARE we say 'Family is for everyone', and I truly believe this. In the past, people with fertility problems often went about creating a family in secret and unorthodox ways, such as by sleeping with someone outside of marriage or covertly adopting a baby. It's always gone on – in biblical times it was called taking a 'handmaid'. Now people can do it safely through IVF. As an example, back in 1997 I helped with the hormonal monitoring of Diane Blood, a young widow who'd fought a legal battle to conceive a child using the stored sperm of her husband who died of meningitis. Before he was ill they'd agreed they wanted to have children, so while he was in a coma doctors extracted sperm from him. Using the sperm to create a baby was a different matter, however, because she didn't have written evidence. This led her to embark on a lengthy legal battle to be allowed to gain access to the sperm. She won, although she still had to go abroad to use it. Over time our children will come to see almost anything as normal and that's no different with IVF. It's a technology that's helped people to create new kinds of families on their own terms.

I know from my own situation how precious that is. I've been lucky to have my four wonderful children, along with a sister and brother-in-law who've always been there for me. And now my eldest, Kate, and her husband have given me my first grandchild; it's shown me how it feels to be part of the flow of generations – the circle of life. A few years ago when my mum was at the grand age of ninety-four, I went up to see her in Liverpool. I knew she hadn't been well and my son Bobby came over to her care home to join me. Finding her in bed and with her breathing heavily laboured, I sat down beside her. She looked pretty bad. What could I do to make her feel better? 'She loves music, Bobby', I said. 'Let's get out my iPod and plug it into the speakers. We'll put her favourite Pavarotti on.'

I held her hand and stroked her face as the notes of *Nessun Dorma* swelled around the room. Her breathing calmed, and a slight smile played around the edges of her mouth. As the song reached its crescendo she went completely still, and I could tell her breathing had stopped. There was a moment's silence. 'I think she's gone', I whispered to Bobby. We were both incredulous that she'd had such an amazing and unexpected death. When the doctor arrived to confirm it he seemed surprised to see me smiling. I said to him, 'Do me a favour. On the death certificate, could you put "death by Pavarotti?"'

I'm sure a lot of people who know me wonder what keeps driving me and why, at the age of sixty-five, I'm not better acquainted with the golf course. Whenever I'm asked, I recount how I once visited Puccini's house in Lucca, Italy. One of the exhibits is a letter he wrote when he discovered he was dying, containing the poignant line: 'Finally, I've realised there will be no more music.' The truth is I don't yet feel able to say 'there will be no more IVF'. In other words, it's just not over. There's too much to do. And despite the toll it takes on my personal life and the people close to me, I can't give it up, not yet.

Being part of pioneering IVF is by necessity to throw oneself into a lions' den of righteous anger and criticism, not to mention the practical difficulties involved. But it's also to be privy to the deepest anguish and fears of the couples I meet, along with their joy and delight when I can make their dreams come true and share in their miracle. Even when I can't help them, I know leaving no stone unturned will alleviate their pain, and this is the fuel that drives my quest. My view has always been that just because something's a challenge, it doesn't mean I won't rise to it. If I can take somebody from despair to hope by giving them a baby, I damn well will.

Author Cited Publications

Appleton TC, Fishel SB. Morphological and elemental analysis of semen from fertile and infertile men used in in vitro fertilisation, J. In Vitro Fert. Emb. Trans. 1, 188, 1984. Fertil. Steril. 42, 191, 1984.

Aslam I, Fishel SB. The use of spermatids for human conception. In: *Signal Transduction in Testicular Cells: Basic and Clinical Aspects*. Hansson et al (eds). Springer-Verlag, Germany. 1996.

Campbell A, Fishel SB, Bowman N, Duffy S, Sedler M, Fontes Lindemann Hickmann C. Modelling a risk classification of aneuploidy in human embryos using non-invasive morphokinetics, *Reprod Biomed Online*, 26, 477–485, 2013a.

Campbell A, Fishel SB, Bowman N, Duffy S, Sedler M, Thornton S. Retrospective analysis of outcomes after IVF using an aneuploidy risk model derived from time-lapse imaging without PGS, *Reprod Biomed Online*, 27, 140–146, 2013b.

Campbell A, Fishel SB, Laedgdsmand M. Aneuploidy is a key causal factor of delays in blastulation detected by time lapse imaging. Author response to 'A cautionary note against aneuploidy risk assessment using time lapse imaging'. *Reprod Biomed Online*, 28, 279–283, 2014.

Cohen J, Edwards RG, Fehilly C, Fishel SB, Hewitt J, Purdy J, Rowland G, Steptoe P, Webster J. In vitro fertilisation: A treatment for male infertility. Fertil. Steril. 43, 422, 1985.

Cohen J, Edwards RG, Fehilly C, Fishel SB, Hewitt J, Rowland G, Steptoe PC, Webster J. Treatment of male infertility by in vitro fertilisation; factors affecting fertilisation and pregnancy. Eur. J. Fertil. Steril. 15, 455, 1985.

Cohen J, Edwards RG, Fehilly C, Fishel SB, Hewitt J, Rowland J. In vitro fertilisation using cryopreserved donor semen in cases where both partners are infertile. Fertil. Steril. 43, 570, 1985.

Cohen J, Fehilly C, Fishel SB, Edwards RG, Hewitt J, Rowland GF, Steptoe PC, Webster J. Male infertility successfully treated by in vitro fertilisation. Lancet i, 1239, 1984.

Cohen J, Simons RF, Edwards RG, Fehilly CB, Fishel SB. Pregnancies following the frozen-storage of expanding human blastocysts. J. In Vitro Fert. Emb. Trans. 2, 59–64, 1985.

Cohen J, Simons RF, Fehilly C, Fishel SB, Edwards RG, Hewitt J, Rowland G, Steptoe PC, Webster J. Birth after replacement of hatching blastocyst cryopreserved at expanded blastocyst stage. Lancet I, 647, 1985.

Cohen J, Simons RF, Fehilly C, Fishel SB, Edwards RG. Cryopreservation of cleaving embryos and expanded blastocysts in the human: A comparative study. Fertil. Steril. 44, 638–639, 1985.

Edwards RG, Fishel SB. The human uterus in the luteal phase and early pregnancy. In: Human Conception In Vitro. Eds: RG Edwards & JM Purdy. Academic Press, 257–288, 1982.

Edwards RG, Fishel SB, Purdy JM. In vitro fertilisation of human eggs; analysis of follicular growth, ovulation and fertilisation. In: Fertilisation of the Human Egg In Vitro, BiologicalBasis and Clinical Application. Eds: HM Beier & HR Lindner Springer–Verlag, Berlin, 169–188, 1983.

Edwards RG, Fishel SB, Cohen J, Fehilly C, Purdy JM, Steptoe PC, Webster J. New physiological considerations resulting from the Experience of fertilisation in vitro. In: Actualities Gynaecologiques, 5th Series, 135 Masson, Paris, 1984a.

Edwards RG, Fishel SB, Cohen J, Fehilly C, Purdy JM. Factors influencing the success of in vitro fertilisation for alleviating human infertility. J. In Vitro Fertil. 1, 1, 1984b.

Edwards RG, Cohen J, Fehilly C, Fishel SB, Hewitt J, Purdy JM, Rowland G, Steptoe PC, Webster J. Observations on the best combination of Clomiphene and Human Menopausal Gonadotrophins for in vitro fertilisation. *Proceedings of the Royal Society, Biology*, 233, 417, 1985.

Fehilly CB, Cohen J, Simons RF, Fishel SB, Edwards RG. Cryopreservations of cleaving embryos and expanded blastocysts in the human: A comparative study. *Fertil. Steril.* 44, 638–644, 1985.

Fishel SB. The mechanism of embryo implantation. In: *Human In Vitro Fertilisation and Early Embryo Development.* Eds: L Bettochi, L Carenza, G Loverro, G Sadurny, CIC, Rome, 225–243, 1984.

Fishel SB. Human in vitro fertilisation and the present state of research on pre–embryonic material, *Int. J. on the Unity of the Sciences*, 2, 173–212, 1988.

Fishel SB. Evidence-based medicine and the role of the National Health Service in assisted reproduction. *Reproductive BioMedicine Online*, 27, 568–569, 2013.

Fishel SB, Antinori S, Jackson P, Johnson J, Lisi F, Chiariello F, Versaci C. Twin birth after subzonal insemination. *The Lancet*, ii, 722, 1990.

Fishel SB, Aslam I, Tesarik J. Spermatid conception: a stage too soon or a time too early? *Human Reproduction*, 11, 1371–1375, 1996.

Fishel SB, Baker DJ, Greer I. LMWH in IVF: Biomarkers and benefits. *Thrombosis Research*, 151, S65–S69, 2017.

Fishel SB, Campbell A, Montgomery S, Smith R, Nice L, Duffy S, Jenner L, Berrisford K, Kellam L, Smith R, D'Cruz I, Beccles A. Live births after embryo selection using morphokinetics versus conventional morphology: a retrospective analysis. *Reprod Biomed Online*, 35, 407–416, 2017.

Fishel SB, Campbell A, Montgomery S, Smith R, Nice L, Duffy S, Jenner L, Berrisford K, Kelham L, Smith R, D'Cruz I, Beccles A. Time-lapse imaging algorithms rank human preimplantation embryos according to their probability to result in a live birth. *Reprod Biomed Online*, 37, 304–313, 2018.

Fishel SB, Cohen J, Fehilly C, Purdy JM, Walters E, Edwards RG. *Factors influencing human embryonic development in vitro.* New York Academy of Sciences, 442, 342–356, 1985.

Fishel SB, Edwards RG. Essentials of fertilisation. In: *Human Conception In Vitro*. Eds: RG Edwards & JM Purdy. Academic Press, 157–179, 1982.

Fishel SB, Edwards RG, Steptoe PC, Purdy JM, Webster J. Establishing and maintaining pregnancy by in vitro fertilisation. In: *In Vitro Fertilisation and Embryo Transfer*. Academic Press, London, 294–304, 1983a.

Fishel SB, Edwards RG, Purdy JM. In vitro fertilisation of human oocytes: factors associated with embryonic development in vitro, replacement of embryos and pregnancy. In: *Fertilisation of the Human Egg In Vitro, Biological Basis and Clinical Application*. Eds: HM Beier & HR Lindner Springer–Verlag, Berlin, 251–270, 1983b.

Fishel SB, Edwards RG, Walters DE. Follicular steroids as prognosticator of successful fertilisation of the human oocyte in vitro.J. Endocrin. 99, 335, 1983c.

Fishel SB, Edwards RG, Evans C. Human chorionic gonadotrophin secreted by pre-implantation embryos cultured in vitro. *Science*, 223, 816, 1984a.

Fishel SB, Edwards RG, Purdy JM. Analysis of 25 infertile patients treated consecutively by in vitro fertilisation at Bourn Hall. Fertil.Steril. 42, 191, 1984b.

Fishel SB, Edwards RG, Purdy JM. Births after a prolonged delay between oocyte recovery and fertilisation in vitro. *Gamete Research* 9, 175, 1984c.

Fishel SB, Edwards RG, Purdy JM, Steptoe PC, Webster J, Walters E, Cohen J, Fehilly C, Hewitt J, Rowland G. Implantation, abortion and birth after in vitro fertilisation using the natural menstrual cycle, or follicular stimulation with Clomiphene Citrate and Human Menopausal Gonadotrophin. J. In Vitro Fert. Emb. Trans. 2, 123–131, 1985a.

Fishel SB, Edwards RG, Purdy JM, Walters DE. Survival of human spermatozoa after preparation for in vitro fertilisation. J. In Vitro Fert. Emb. Trans. 2, 233–235, 1985b.

Fishel SB, Green S, Bishop M, Thornton S, Hunter A, Fleming S, Al-Hassan S. Pregnancy after intracytoplasmic injection of a spermatid in the human. *The Lancet*, 345, 1641–1642, 1995.

Fishel, SB, Greer I, Baker D, Elson J, Ragunath M, Atkinson G, Shaker A, Omar A, Kazem R, Beccles A. Precision medicine in assisted conception: A multi center observational treatment cohort study of the annexin A5 M2 haplotype as a biomarker for antithrombotic treatment to improve pregnancy outcome. Ebiomedicine, 10, 298–304, 2016.

Fishel SB, Jackson P. Follicular stimulation for high-tech pregnancies: are we playing it safe? B.M.J. 299, 309–311, 1989.

Fishel SB, Lisi F, Rinaldi L, Green S, Hunter A, Dowell K, Thornton S. Systematic Examination of immobilizing spermatozoa before intracytoplasmic sperm injection in the human. Human Reproduction, 10, 497–500, 1995.

Fishel SB, Patel R, Lytollis A, Robinson J, Smedley M, Smith P, Cameron C, Thornton S, Dowell K, Atkinson G, Shaker A, Lowe P, Kazem R, Brett S, Fox A. A multicentre study of the clinical relevance of screening IVF patients for carrier status of the annexin A5 M2 haplotype. Reprod Biomed Online, 29, 80–87, 2014.

Fishel SB, Symonds, EM (eds). In Vitro Fertilisation: Past, Present, Future. IRL Press, Oxford, 1986.

Fishel SB, Timson J, Lisi F, Rinaldi L. Subzonal insemination and zona breaching techniques for assisted fertilisation. In: Gamete and Embryo Micromanipulation in Human Reproduction. Eds: SB Fishel & EM Symonds. Edward Arnold Publishers, 79–97, 1993.

Fishel SB, Walters DE, Yodyinguad V, Edwards RG. Time-dependent motility changes of human spermatozoa after preparation for in vitro fertilization. J. In Vitro Fert. Emb. Trans. 2, 233–235, 1985.

Forman R, Cohen J, Fehilly C, Fishel SB, Edwards RG. The application of the Zona–Free Hamster Egg Test for the prognosis of human in vitro fertilisation. J. In Vitro Fert. Emb. Trans. 1, 166, 1984.

Forman R, Fishel SB, Edwards RG, Walters E. Influence of transient hyperprolactinaemia on in vitro fertilisation in the human. J. Clin. Endocrin. Meta. 60, 517–522, 1985.

Hewitt J, Cohen J, Fehilly C, Rowland G, Steptoe PC, Webster J, Edwards RG, Fishel SB. Seminal bacterial pathogens and in vitro fertilisation. J. In Vitro Fert. Emb. Trans. 2, 105–106, 1985.

Scobie G, Woodroffe B, Fishel SB, Kalsheker N. Identification of the five most common cystic fibrosis mutations in single cells using a rapid and specific differential amplification system. *Molecular Human Reproduction*, 2, 203–207, 1996.

Steptoe PC, Edwards RG, Webster J, Fishel SB, Cohen J, Fehilly C, Hewitt J, Rowland G, Walters E. Observations on 533 clinical pregnancies and 242 births after in vitro fertilisation. *American Journal of Obstetrics & Gynaecology*; 153, 1985.

Steptoe PC, Webster J, Fishel SB, Edwards RG, Purdy, J. Clinical facets of in vitro fertilisation in the human. In: *In Vitro Fertilisation and Embryo Transfer*. Academic Press, London, 306–314, 1983.

Wikland M, Fishel SB, Hamberger L. Novel aspects on ultrasound guided follicular aspiration. In: *Human In Vitro Fertilization*; INSERM Symposium No. 24. Eds: J Testart & R Frydman Elsevier Science, Amsterdam, 45–52, 1985.

Wikland M, Fishel SB, Hamberger L. *Oocyte recovery by sonographic techniques*. International Society on Human In-Vitro Fertilisation, Montreal, Canada, 1984.

About the Author

Professor Simon Fishel is one of the world's leading IVF experts. In the 1970s and '80s he worked closely with Robert Edwards and Patrick Steptoe, the duo who first successfully pioneered conception through IVF, leading to the birth of Louise Brown in 1978. After gaining his doctorate at Cambridge he continued his work with the pair as Deputy Scientific Director of Bourn Hall, the world's first independent IVF clinic. While he was there, he helped organise the very first IVF conference.

During his forty years leading the field in assisted reproduction, Simon has spearheaded numerous innovations, including sperm injection technology to enable men to father their own children. He was also the first in the UK to attempt a saviour sibling conception, to develop chromosome screening for pre-implantation embryos, and to use embryo vitrification to make incubation more effective and affordable. More recently he published his organisation's ground-breaking use of time-lapse imaging technology for improving IVF success rates, called CAREmaps. His mission to keep improving IVF has led him to travel all over the world, teaching other practitioners and treating patients. As part of this aim he set up the world's first Master's degree course in IVF in order to raise standards in global practice.

In the course of his career Simon has written over 200 scientific papers and published a number of books. He's received awards from countries such as Japan, Austria, South Africa, and Italy, and has advised numerous international governments including the Vatican. He's an elected Fellow of the Royal Society of Biology (FRSB).

As a born and bred Liverpudlian, in 1994, Simon was delighted (and somewhat embarrassed) to be voted one of Liverpool's 'Top ten living legends', and in 2009 received an Honorary Fellowship from Liverpool John Moores' University for his 'outstanding contributions to humanity and science in the field of fertility treatment, including embryology and IVF'. He was also placed at number ten in the '100 Hottest Health Gurus' by women's health and wellbeing magazine *Top Santé* in its September 2013 issue.

In 1997 he founded what is now the UK's largest chain of IVF clinics, CARE Fertility Group, and ten years later won the Ernst and Young Entrepreneur of the Year Award (regional winner). Today, as President, he also continues to head up CARE's research programme and is raising greater awareness for secondary infertility through his charity The Rachel Foundation. His next complementary venture is ProFaM, a company set up for the dual purpose of improving women's health by not only preserving fertility but by naturally delaying the menopause.

Acknowledgements

'Life's challenges are not supposed to paralyse you, they're supposed to help you discover who you are', said Bernice Johnson Reagon. This is true, but we all need support.

Throughout my life I've been privileged to be surrounded by warm-hearted, caring, and supportive family, friends, and colleagues. I've also been blessed with understanding and special children, Kate, Matt, Bobs, and Sav, who have often come second to my work but who have always been remembered and loved. Now they're adults in their own rights, each with a unique spirit of their own. For them I wish nothing less than to feel as professionally fulfilled as I have been. To them I express my immense gratitude and love.

I'd like to give special thanks to some colleagues who've accompanied me on my journey, and who've courageously exemplified how to look after those who've put their faith in them. John Webster, who was with me at the beginning and who continues to spend time with me, but who hasn't yet got me on the golf course. My admiration for him as a doctor remains unsurpassed after all these decades and I'm enormously proud that our central clinic is named John Webster House. Ali, Judy, Louise, Kathryn, and Ken, who were there in the early days of Nurture: what a privilege it is to work with them still. And of course Simon, who still blames me for his grey hair, but now he's retired with a new career, my sympathy has somewhat dissipated! And Wanda, who for twenty-six years has not only understood what I want to achieve, but with her marvellous communication skills, enormous compassion for patients, and utter dedication to the cause, has conveyed to the wider world how important our 'breakthrough babies' are. They're all miracles.

This book would never have come into existence without the wonderful and professional support of Ginny Carter. It was one thing to think that someday I might put my thoughts on paper and that maybe those thoughts would be turned into some kind of book. But in truth, when I assumed I'd wait until my retirement to do this, I realised I may never get the chance let alone have the capability. On recommendation I found Ginny, and in a remarkably short space of time she enabled me to turn my verbosity and complex view of how the last forty years has gone into something I could never have achieved on my own. I shall be forever grateful for her skill.

And last but certainly not least Maggie, who knew me in those early IVF days when I scrabbled and fought for each and every case, working long days and even longer nights, juggling clinical cases and trying to understand the basic nature of the science and what it would come to mean to humanity; and who all these years later has become part of the book of my life. To her I say simply, there's still so much more to share.